Update in Cancer Screening

Editors

ROBERT A. SMITH
KEVIN C. OEFFINGER

MEDICAL CLINICS
OF NORTH AMERICA

www.medical.theclinics.com

Consulting Editor
JACK ENDE

November 2020 • Volume 104 • Number 6

ELSEVIER

1600 John F. Kennedy Boulevard • Suite 1800 • Philadelphia, Pennsylvania, 19103-2899

http://www.theclinics.com

MEDICAL CLINICS OF NORTH AMERICA Volume 104, Number 6
November 2020 ISSN 0025-7125, ISBN-13: 978-0-323-78953-0

Editor: Katerina Heidhausen
Developmental Editor: Nick Henderson

Medical Clinics of North America (ISSN 0025-7125) is published bimonthly by Elsevier Inc., 360 Park Avenue South, New York, NY 10010-1710. Months of publication are January, March, May, July, September, and November. Business and editorial offices: 1600 John F. Kennedy Boulevard, Suite 1800, Philadelphia, PA 19103-2899. Periodicals postage paid at New York, NY, and additional mailing offices. Subscription prices are USD $295.00 per year (US individuals), $654.00 per year (US institutions), $100.00 per year (US Students), $353.00 per year (Canadian individuals), $850.00 per year (Canadian institutions), $200.00 per year (foreign students), $100.00 per year for (Canadian students), $422.00 per year (foreign individuals), and $850.00 per year (foreign institutions). To receive student/resident rate, orders must be accompanied by name of affiliated institution, date of term, and the signature of program/residency coordinator on institution letterhead. Orders will be billed at individual rate until proof of status is received. Foreign air speed delivery is included in all Clinics' subscription prices. All prices are subject to change without notice. **POSTMASTER:** Send address changes to *Medical Clinics of North America*, Elsevier Health Sciences Division, Subscription Customer Service, 3251 Riverport Lane, Maryland Heights, MO 63043. **Customer Service: Telephone: 1-800-654-2452** (U.S. and Canada); **1-314-447-8871** (outside U.S. and Canada). **Fax: 314-447-8029. E-mail: journalscustomerserviceusa@ elsevier.com** (for print support); **journalsonlinesupport-usa@elsevier.com** (for online support).

Reprints. For copies of 100 or more of articles in this publication, please contact the Commercial Reprints Department, Elsevier Inc., 360 Park Avenue South, New York, NY 10010-1710. Tel.: 212-633-3874; Fax: 212-633-3820; E-mail: reprints@elsevier.com.

Medical Clinics of North America is also published in Spanish by McGraw-Hill Interamericana Editores S. A., P.O. Box 5-237, 06500 Mexico, D.F., Mexico.

Medical Clinics of North America is covered in *MEDLINE/PubMed (Index Medicus), Current Contents, ASCA, Excerpta Medica, Science Citation Index,* and *ISI/BIOMED.*

PROGRAM OBJECTIVE

The goal of the *Medical Clinics of North America* is to keep practicing physicians up to date with current clinical practice by providing timely articles reviewing the state of the art in patient care.

TARGET AUDIENCE

All practicing physicians and other healthcare professionals.

LEARNING OBJECTIVES

Upon completion of this activity, participants will be able to:

1. Review cancer screening recommendations for older adults, the evidence regarding breast cancer screening for average risk women, colorectal screening modalities, lung cancer screening practices, effective strategies for cervical cancer prevention, and the current state of the evidence for prostate cancer screening and early detection.
2. Explain how the evaluation of various cancer screening methods, variation in guideline quality and development, and widespread implementation of cancer screening affect cancer detection and prevention.
3. Discuss the impact a system of organized cancer screening could make in addressing the challenges of risk assessment, informed/shared decision making, reminders for screening, and tracking adherence to screening recommendations.

ACCREDITATION

The Elsevier Office of Continuing Medical Education (EOCME) is accredited by the Accreditation Council for Continuing Medical Education (ACCME) to provide continuing medical education for physicians.

The EOCME designates this journal-based CME activity for a maximum of 10 *AMA PRA Category 1 Credit*(s)™. Physicians should claim only the credit commensurate with the extent of their participation in the activity.

All other healthcare professionals requesting continuing education credit for this enduring material will be issued a certificate of participation.

DISCLOSURE OF CONFLICTS OF INTEREST

The EOCME assesses conflict of interest with its instructors, faculty, planners, and other individuals who are in a position to control the content of CME activities. All relevant conflicts of interest that are identified are thoroughly vetted by EOCME for fair balance, scientific objectivity, and patient care recommendations. EOCME is committed to providing its learners with CME activities that promote improvements or quality in healthcare and not a specific proprietary business or a commercial interest.

The planning committee, staff, authors and editors listed below have identified no financial relationships or relationships to products or devices they or their spouse/life partner have with commercial interest related to the content of this CME activity:

Sigrid V. Carlsson, MD, PhD, MPH; Regina Chavous-Gibson, MSN, RN; Michael Conner, MD; Stephen W. Duffy, BSc, MSc, Cstat; Jack Ende, MD, MACP; Terresa J. Eun, AB; Katerina Heidhausen; Nick Henderson; Thomas Houston, MD; Albert Jang, MD; Ashwin A. Kotwal, MD, MS; Christoph I. Lee, MD, MS; Constance D. Lehman, MD, PhD; Eric M. Montminy, MD; Anand K. Narayan, MD, PhD; Kevin C. Oeffinger, MD; Rebecca B. Perkins, MD, MSc; Robert A. Smith, PhD; Jeyanthi Surendrakumar; Louise C. Walter, MD; Richard Wender, MD; Andrew M.D. Wolf, MD.

The planning committee, staff, authors and editors listed below have identified financial relationships or relationships to products or devices they or their spouse/life partner have with commercial interest related to the content of this CME activity:

Jordan J. Karlitz, MD: a consultant/advisor for Exact Sciences Corporation, a consultant/advisor and speakers bureau for Myriad Genetics, Inc., and owns stock in Gastro Girl.

Andrew J. Vickers, PhD: owns stock and earns royalties from OPKO Health, Inc.

UNAPPROVED/OFF-LABEL USE DISCLOSURE

The EOCME requires CME faculty to disclose to the participants;

1. When products or procedures being discussed are off-label, unlabelled, experimental, and/or investigational (not US Food and Drug Administration [FDA] approved); and
2. Any limitations on the information presented, such as data that are preliminary or that represent ongoing research, interim analyses, and/or unsupported opinions. Faculty may discuss information about

pharmaceutical agents that is outside of FDA-approved labelling. This information is intended solely for CME and is not intended to promote off-label use of these medications. If you have any questions, contact the medical affairs department of the manufacturer for the most recent prescribing information.

TO ENROLL

To enroll in the *Medical Clinics of North America* Continuing Medical Education program, call customer service at 1-800-654-2452 or sign up online at http://www.theclinics.com/home/cme. The CME program is available to subscribers for an additional annual fee of USD 300.00.

METHOD OF PARTICIPATION

In order to claim credit, participants must complete the following;
1. Complete enrolment as indicated above.
2. Read the activity.
3. Complete the CME Test and Evaluation. Participants must achieve a score of 70% on the test. All CME Tests and Evaluations must be completed online.

CME INQUIRIES/SPECIAL NEEDS

For all CME inquiries or special needs, please contact elsevierCME@elsevier.com.

MEDICAL CLINICS OF NORTH AMERICA

SERIES OF RELATED INTEREST

Physician Assistant Clinics
https://www.physicianassistant.theclinics.com/
Primary Care: Clinics in Office Practice
https://www.primarycare.theclinics.com/

Contributors

CONSULTING EDITOR

JACK ENDE, MD, MACP
The Schaeffer Professor of Medicine, Perelman School of Medicine of the University of Pennsylvania, Philadelphia, Pennsylvania, USA

EDITORS

ROBERT A. SMITH, PhD
Senior Vice President, Cancer Screening, Cancer Prevention and Early Detection Department, Director, Center for Cancer Screening, American Cancer Society, Atlanta, Georgia, USA

KEVIN C. OEFFINGER, MD
Professor of Medicine, Director, Center for Onco-Primary Care, Director, Supportive Care and Survivorship Center, Duke Cancer Institute, Duke University School of Medicine, Durham, North Carolina, USA

AUTHORS

SIGRID V. CARLSSON, MD, PhD, MPH
Assistant Attending, Department of Surgery (Urology Service), Department of Epidemiology and Biostatistics, Memorial Sloan Kettering Cancer Center, New York, New York, USA; Department of Urology, Institute of Clinical Sciences, Sahlgrenska Academy at University of Gothenburg, Gothenburg, Sweden

MICHAEL CONNER, MD
Internal Medicine Resident, Department of Internal Medicine, Tulane University School of Medicine, New Orleans, Louisiana, USA

STEPHEN W. DUFFY, MSc
Professor of Cancer Screening, Wolfson Institute of Preventive Medicine, Queen Mary University of London, London, United Kingdom

TERRESA J. EUN, AB
Doctoral Candidate, Department of Sociology, Stanford University, Stanford, California, USA

THOMAS HOUSTON, MD
Adjunct Professor, Department of Family Medicine, The Ohio State University College of Medicine, Columbus, Ohio, USA

ALBERT JANG, MD
Internal Medicine Resident, Department of Internal Medicine, Tulane University School of Medicine, New Orleans, Louisiana, USA

JORDAN J. KARLITZ, MD
Associate Professor of Medicine, Division of Gastroenterology, Southeastern Louisiana Veterans Healthcare System, Tulane University School of Medicine, New Orleans, Louisiana, USA

ASHWIN A. KOTWAL, MD, MS
Division of Geriatrics, Department of Medicine, University of California, San Francisco, Geriatrics, Palliative, and Extended Care Service Line, San Francisco Veterans Affairs Medical Center, San Francisco, California, USA

CHRISTOPH I. LEE, MD, MS
Professor, Department of Radiology, Adjunct Professor, Department of Health Services, Director, Northwest Screening and Cancer Outcomes Research Enterprise, University of Washington, Seattle, Washington, USA

CONSTANCE D. LEHMAN, MD, PhD
Professor of Radiology, Harvard Medical School, Chief of Breast Imaging and Co-Director of Avon Breast Center, Massachusetts General Hospital, Boston, Massachusetts, USA

ERIC M. MONTMINY, MD
Gastroenterology Fellow, Division of Gastroenterology, Tulane University School of Medicine, New Orleans, Louisiana, USA

ANAND K. NARAYAN, MD, PhD
Assistant Professor, Radiology, Massachusetts General Hospital, Boston, Massachusetts, USA

KEVIN C. OEFFINGER, MD
Professor of Medicine, Director, Center for Onco-Primary Care, Director, Supportive Care and Survivorship Center, Duke Cancer Institute, Duke University School of Medicine, Durham, North Carolina, USA

REBECCA B. PERKINS, MD, MSc
Associate Professor, Department of Obstetrics and Gynecology, Boston University School of Medicine, Boston Medical Center, Boston, Massachusetts, USA

ROBERT A. SMITH, PhD
Senior Vice President, Cancer Screening, Cancer Prevention and Early Detection Department, Director, Center for Cancer Screening, American Cancer Society, Atlanta, Georgia, USA

ANDREW J. VICKERS, PhD
Attending, Department of Epidemiology and Biostatistics, Memorial Sloan Kettering Cancer Center, New York, New York, USA

LOUISE C. WALTER, MD
Division of Geriatrics, Department of Medicine, University of California, San Francisco, Geriatrics, Palliative, and Extended Care Service Line, San Francisco Veterans Affairs Medical Center, San Francisco, California, USA

RICHARD WENDER, MD
Chair, Family Medicine and Community Health, University of Pennsylvania, Philadelphia, Pennsylvania, USA

ANDREW M.D. WOLF, MD
Professor, Department of Medicine, University of Virginia School of Medicine, Charlottesville, Virginia, USA

Contents

The burden of cancer in the United States is substantial, providing important opportunity and obligation for primary care clinicians to promote cancer prevention and early detection. Without a system of organized
screening to support reminders and follow-up of cancer screening, primary care clinicians face challenges in addressing risk assessment,
informed/shared decision making, reminders for screening, and tracking
adherence to screening recommendations. Tools exist for collecting information about family history, tracking screening adherence, and reminding
patients when they are due for screening, and strategies exist for making
cancer prevention and early detection an office policy and delegating roles
and responsibilities to office staff.

Cancer screening uses many investigative procedures, and different
screening programs and methods have different objectives. For example,
mammography aims to detect breast cancer at an earlier stage when successful treatment is more likely, whereas colonoscopy is aimed primarily at
detecting adenomas in the colon and removing them, thus preventing
them from progressing to cancer at all. Evaluation has different objectives,
including proof of principle, checking that screening services are delivering
the desired clinical outcome, technical quality control of the investigation
procedures. All necessitate a range of tools for evaluation. We review
these tools, with particular attention to appropriate outcome measures.

Clinicians and the public have always depended on expert advice to guide
clinical practice. However, since the 1970s, a growing emphasis on
evidence-based medicine has led to clinical practice guidelines being
less expert based and increasingly evidence based with judgments about
the balance between the two. Because the existence of standards for
guidelines development is no guarantee that a guideline will be trustworthy, tools and instruments have been developed to measure the

degree to which a guideline has been developed with rigorous adherence to methodology, and has not been influenced by conflicts of interest.

Screening for cancer has contributed to substantial reductions in death from several cancers and is one of the most cost-effective preventive interventions in all of health care. In the United States, primary care clinicians, their clinical teams, and the systems in which they work are primarily responsible for ensuring that screening occurs. In order to achieve the highest possible population-wide screening rates, primary care clinicians must embrace the responsibility to screen their entire enrolled patient population, institute several overarching general approaches to screening, and implement a combination of evidence-based interventions.

Cancer screening decisions in older adults can be complex due to the unclear cancer-specific mortality benefits of screening and several known harms including false positives, overdiagnosis, and procedural complications from downstream diagnostic interventions. In this review, we provide a framework for individualized cancer screening decisions among older adults, involving accounting for overall health and life expectancy, individual values, and the risks and benefits of specific cancer screening tests. We then discuss strategies for effective communication of recommendations during clinical visits that are considered more effective, easy to understand, and acceptable by older adults and clinicians.

Among women, breast cancer is the most commonly diagnosed cancer and the leading cause of cancer-related death in the world. The purpose of this article is to review the evidence regarding breast cancer screening for average-risk women. The review primarily focuses on mammographic screening but also reviews clinical breast examinations, emerging screening technologies, and opportunities to build consensus. Wherever possible, the review relies on published systematic reviews, meta-analyses, and guidelines from three major societies (US Preventive Services Task Force, American College of Radiology, and the American Cancer Society) to reflect a range of evidence-based perspectives regarding mammographic screening.

Colorectal cancer screening is essential to detect and remove premalignant lesions to prevent the development of colorectal cancer. Multiple screening modalities are available, including colonoscopy and stool-based testing. Colonoscopy remains the gold standard for detection and removal of premalignant colorectal lesions. Screening guidelines by the American Cancer Society now recommend initiating screening for all average-risk adults at 45 years old. Family history of colorectal cancer, other cancers, and advanced colon polyps are strong risk factors that must be considered in order to implement earlier testing. Epidemiologic studies continue to show disparities in colorectal cancer incidence and mortality and wide variability in screening rates.

Thomas Houston

Lung cancer screening with low-dose computed tomography provides an opportunity to save lives by early detection of the deadliest cancer in the United States. Uptake of lung cancer screening has been quite low but may be improving. Clinician and patient education, integration of lung cancer screening protocols into electronic medical records, support for shared decision making and tobacco cessation, and improved communication between referral centers and clinicians are all important areas for improvement for lung cancer screening to reach its potential in improving morbidity and mortality from lung cancer.

Sigrid V. Carlsson and Andrew J. Vickers

This article gives an overview of the current state of the evidence for prostate cancer early detection with prostate-specific antigen (PSA) and summarizes current recommendations from guideline groups. The article reviews the global public health burden and risk factors for prostate cancer with clinical implications as screening tools. Screening studies, novel biomarkers, and MRI are discussed. The article outlines 7 key practice points for primary care physicians and provides a simple schema for facilitating shared decision-making conversations.

Terresa J. Eun and Rebecca B. Perkins

The most effective strategy for cervical cancer prevention involves vaccination against human papillomavirus (HPV) infection during adolescence followed by screening during adulthood. HPV vaccination before sexual debut can prevent HPV infections, precancers, and cancers. HPV vaccination of sexually active populations does not prevent cancer. Screening is critical to prevent cancer between the ages of 25 and 65. Screening with HPV testing or cotesting is more effective than Pap testing alone. Ensuring adequate screening at ages 45-65 may prevent cervical cancer among elderly women. Most cervical cancers at all ages occur among unscreened or underscreened women.

Foreword
Cancer Screening: Finding the Path Forward

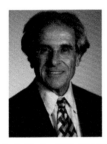

Jack Ende, MD, MACP
Consulting Editor

Nothing should be more straightforward than screening for cancer, or so one might think. After all, is not early detection of cancer consistently associated with better outcomes? Are not serologic, endoscopic, and radiologic tests always objective and accurate. Decisions for cancer screening should be straightforward, but, of course, they are not. Why not?

First, there are harms associated with screening. These include the costs associated with screening protocols, the medical complications of the screening procedures and the treatments that may follow, and the psychological distress that can arise from knowing that one has an illness such as cancer, particularly if early treatment is not advantageous.

Second, there remains a disquieting lack of consensus on the most effective screening tests, the optimal interval for screening, and the threshold for a positive result. Add to that the variations in test interpretation, the operating characteristics of tests (sensitivity and specificity), and the panoply of socioeconomic, cultural, racial, genetic, and behavioral issues, that bear upon how and when to screen patients and populations. Decisions regarding cancer screening are complex and nuanced. But these decisions are critical, as doctors and patients must decide how to screen for malignancy and what to do with the results.

This issue of *Medical Clinics of North America* provides a sophisticated, up-to-date overview of cancer screening. It includes integrative articles on the criteria by which screening recommendations can be assessed, the strategies by which those recommendations can be implemented, and the standards that inform the formulation of screening guidelines. Information specific for screening elderly populations completes the integrative articles. Then, updated recommendations based upon the best available evidence, for screening for some of the most important and common malignancies– breast, colon, lung, cervical, and prostate cancers– are provided.

Med Clin N Am 104 (2020) xiii–xiv
https://doi.org/10.1016/j.mcna.2020.08.011
0025-7125/20/© 2020 Published by Elsevier Inc.

medical.theclinics.com

Experienced clinicians, of course, are prepared to handle less-than-straightforward recommendations and certainly that applies to cancer screening. The data regarding cancer screening are not always concordant; recommendations vary, and they change. Patient preferences amplify that complexity. But, in this issue, through the diligent work of the guest editors, Drs Robert Smith and Kevin Oeffinger, and their expert authors, readers will find the most valuable, current information available, information they will need to help guide their patients through the complex yet critical decision-making process of screening for cancer.

Jack Ende, MD, MACP
The Schaeffer Professor of Medicine
Perelman School of Medicine of the
University of Pennsylvania
5033 West Gates Pavilion
3400 Spruce Street
Philadelphia, PA 19104, USA

E-mail address:
jack.ende@pennmedicine.upenn.edu

Preface

Cancer Screening in Primary Care: So Much Progress, So Much Left to Do

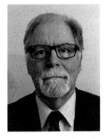 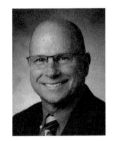

Robert A. Smith, PhD   Kevin C. Oeffinger, MD
Editors

In this update on cancer screening, it is sobering to realize that the first comprehensive evaluation of cancer screening guidelines took place 40 years ago when the American Cancer Society (ACS) commissioned Dr David Eddy and his colleagues to apply the principles of evidence-based medicine to the ACS' recommendations for the early detection of cancer.[1] Shortly thereafter in 1984, the US Preventive Services Task Force was commissioned and charged with bringing evidence-based medicine to the evaluation of common interventions in the primary care setting, and 5 years later, issued its first report on 169 preventive health interventions, including several cancer screening tests.[2] Over the years, these 2 organizations and others have regularly updated guidance to clinicians and the public, and although there have been differences, they always have shared more in common than they differed. Also important, over the past several decades, guideline development methodology has steadily evolved to promote rigor, transparency, and the obligation to address not only the benefits of cancer screening but also the limitations and potential harms.[3,4]

The importance and value of regularly updated evidence-based cancer screening recommendations are overshadowed by a simple reality. The potential to avert disability and premature deaths from those cancers for which we have evidence for the efficacy of screening is dependent on the quality of the screening process and protocol, and regular attendance by the target population. All screening guidelines are based on an assessment of population-based benefit, a starting age is based on the underlying prevalence of disease, a stopping age is based on the likelihood of benefit in the context of longevity, and screening intervals are based on what is known about the tumor's detectable preclinical phase. However, the guidance and the infrastructure do not benefit the adult who does not attend screening; the potential to benefit from

Med Clin N Am 104 (2020) xv–xvii
https://doi.org/10.1016/j.mcna.2020.09.002
0025-7125/20/© 2020 Published by Elsevier Inc.

screening may be less in the adult who attends irregularly and is diagnosed with an advanced cancer after a lapse in attendance, and regular attendance can be an empty exercise if a detectable cancer is missed due to poor quality. Thankfully, the importance of quality assurance in cancer screening has received considerable attention, and although shortcomings in quality still exist, the average adults undergoing screening can be confident that they are receiving a good-quality examination. This leaves lack of attendance and irregular attendance as the principal factors contributing to the unfulfilled potential of cancer screening.

Early on, there was growing recognition of the critically important role of the referring physician's recommendation,[5] the importance of that recommendation being accompanied by informed and shared decision making,[6] and the importance of office systems and policies[7] that would overlay principles of population-based medicine to ensure timely cancer screening and follow-up beyond what is achievable under a model of opportunistic screening, for instance, when referrals to screening depend on encounters with health services, where, for a variety of reasons, a referral may or may not take place.[8] Insufficient time, and the nature of the encounter are common reasons screening referrals don't take place, and thus, it should come as no surprise that patients who have had a preventive health examination are much more likely to report recent cancer screening than patients who only have encounters for acute and chronic complaints.[9] It also is well established that access to cancer screening and screening outcomes in the United States vary by race/ethnicity, education, health literacy, income, occupation, insurance status, geography, and so forth,[10] and that institutional barriers are deeply rooted in the health care system as well.[11] However, most unscreened and underscreened adults who would undergo screening have health insurance, and only need the focused, sometimes relentless, advice from their provider to motivate them to attend screening. For this to happen, practice settings must know who among their patient panel is due for screening, and it must be a practice policy and priority that as many patients who will choose to undergo screening receive regular screening according to the recommendations from expert groups. Most adults will not develop the cancers for which screening is recommended. However, if they do, regular screening will give them the best chance to prevent a precancerous lesion from becoming invasive, to avoid a diagnosis of advanced disease, and to avert a premature death.

In this issue you will find up-to-date advice from leading experts in cancer screening. It has been our pleasure to assemble them to contribute to this issue of *Medical Clinics of North America*, and we are deeply grateful that they agreed to share their wisdom. We also are grateful to the editorial team for support.

Robert A. Smith, PhD
American Cancer Society
250 Williams Street, NW, Suite 600
Atlanta, GA 30303, USA

Kevin C. Oeffinger, MD
Center for Onco-Primary Care
Duke Cancer Institute
2424 Erwin Drive, Suite 601
Durham, NC, USA

E-mail addresses:
robert.smith@cancer.org (R.A. Smith)
kevin.oeffinger@duke.edu (K.C. Oeffinger)

REFERENCES

1. Eddy D. ACS report on the cancer-related health checkup. CA Cancer J Clin 1980;30(4):193–240.
2. U.S. Preventive Services Task Force. Guide to clinical preventive services: an assessment of the effectiveness of 169 interventions. Baltimore (MD): Williams & Wilkins; 1989. p. 1–294.
3. Institute of Medicine. Clinical practice guidelines we can trust. Washington, DC: National Academies Press; 2011. p. 1–266.
4. Institute of Medicine. Finding what works in health care: standards for systematic reviews. Washington, DC: National Academies Press; 2011. p. 1–317.
5. Peterson EB, Ostroff JS, DuHamel KN, et al. Impact of provider-patient communication on cancer screening adherence: a systematic review. Prev Med 2016; 93:96–105.
6. Woolf SH, Krist AH, Lafata JE, et al. Engaging patients in decisions about cancer screening: exploring the decision journey through the use of a patient portal. Am J Prev Med 2018;54(2):237–47.
7. Brandzel SD, Bowles EJA, Wieneke A, et al. Cancer screening reminders: addressing the spectrum of patient preferences. Perm J 2017;21:17–051.
8. Miles A, Cockburn J, Smith RA, et al. A perspective from countries using organized screening programs. Cancer 2004;101(5 Suppl):1201–13.
9. Fenton JJ, Cai Y, Weiss NS, et al. Delivery of cancer screening: how important is the preventive health examination? Arch Intern Med 2007;167(6):580–5.
10. Green BL, Davis JL, Rivers D, et al. Cancer health disparities. In: Alberts D, Hell L, editors. Fundamentals of cancer prevention. Switzerland: Springer; 2019. p. 199–246.
11. Paradies Y, Truong M, Priest N. A systematic review of the extent and measurement of healthcare provider racism. J Gen Intern Med 2014;29(2):364–87.

The Importance of Cancer Screening

Robert A. Smith, PhD[a],*, Kevin C. Oeffinger, MD[b]

KEYWORDS

- Early detection • Cancer screening • Guidelines • Cancer screening rates • Survival

KEY POINTS

- Cancer is a leading cause of death in the world and the leading cause of premature death in the United States.
- A common feature of many cancers is that outcomes generally are more favorable when the disease is detected at a localized stage.
- Cancer screening is defined as testing to detect presymptomatic or undetected symptomatic disease in a population in order to reduce the incidence rate of advanced disease.
- Because there is no system of organized screening across the United States, primary care plays a pivotal role in discussions with patients and referrals to cancer screening.
- Primary care providers are encouraged to support the development of systems in their practice setting to facilitate high rates of adherence to cancer screening recommendations.

INTRODUCTION

A common feature of many cancers is that outcomes generally are more favorable when a disease is detected at a localized stage, and treatment is initiated early in the disease's natural history. This observation, which is evident in survival statistics, has motivated researchers and clinicians to develop and evolve screening technologies to detect occult and early symptomatic disease and to establish methodological principles and study designs to evaluate the efficacy of offering a screening test to an asymptomatic population. If supporting evidence for the value of screening is convincing and benefits are judged to outweigh harms, authoritative bodies are motivated to issue guidelines and recommendations and to establish supporting policies promoting the uptake of cancer screening.

[a] Cancer Prevention and Early Detection Department, Center for Cancer Screening, American Cancer Society, 250 Williams Street, Northwest, Suite 600, Atlanta, GA 30303, USA; [b] Center for Onco-Primary Care, Supportive Care and Survivorship Center, Duke Cancer Institute, Duke University School of Medicine, 2424 Erwin Drive, Suite 601, Durham, NC 27705, USA
* Corresponding author.
E-mail address: robert.smith@cancer.org

Med Clin N Am 104 (2020) 919–938
https://doi.org/10.1016/j.mcna.2020.08.008
0025-7125/20/© 2020 Elsevier Inc. All rights reserved.

medical.theclinics.com

Cancer screening is defined as testing to detect presymptomatic or undetected symptomatic disease in a population in order to reduce the incidence rate of advanced disease and initiate treatment earlier. For some cancers, detecting and treating precursor lesions also is a goal, thus also contributing to reduced morbidity and mortality through reductions in the incidence of invasive disease. When considering cervical cancer screening, the detection of precancerous lesions is the primary goal of screening, and, for colorectal cancer screening, all colorectal cancer screening tests are evaluated for their potential to detect invasive disease and advanced adenomas. Today, the health systems of most developed nations and many developing nations support screening the population for 1 or more of the common cancers.[1,2]

THE BURDEN OF CANCER

Globally, the burden of cancer is substantial and growing. The International Agency for Research on Cancer (IARC) estimates that in 2018 there were approximately 18.1 million new diagnoses of cancer (**Figs. 1** and **2**), approximately 9.5 million deaths (**Figs. 3** and **4**), and, for the most recent 5-year period, an estimated prevalence of approximately 43.8 million individuals living with cancer.[3] By 2040, IARC estimates that the incidence of cancer will have risen to 29.5 million new cases in that year.[4] Cancer is the first or second leading cause of premature death (deaths occurring at ages 30–69 years) in 134 of 183 countries, and over time the burden of disease is expected to grow in low-income to middle-income countries.[5] Of the 6 most common cancers diagnosed each year worldwide (lung, breast, colorectal, prostate, stomach, and cervix), 5 are cancers in which early detection tests have proved efficacy.[6]

In the United States, the burden of cancer also is substantial. In 2020, an estimated 1.8 million Americans will be diagnosed with invasive cancer, and 606,520 will die from cancer.[7] The estimated number of invasive cancers expected in 2020 excludes basal and squamous cell skin cancers, of which more than 5 million new cases occur

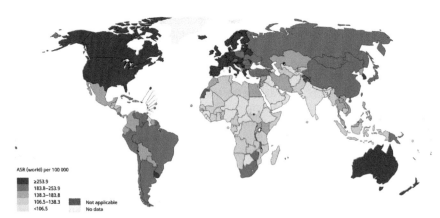

Fig. 1. Estimated age-standardized incidence rates (world) in 2018, all cancers, both sexes, all ages. All rights reserved. The designations employed and the presentation of the material in this publication do not imply the expression of any opinion whatsoever on the part of the World Health Organization/IARC concerning the legal status of any country, territory, city, or area or of its authorities, or concerning the delimitation of its frontiers or boundaries. Dotted and dashed lines on maps represent approximate borderlines for which there may not yet be full agreement. (Data source: GLOBOCAN 2018 Graph production: IARC (http://gco.iarc.fr/today) World Health Organization.)

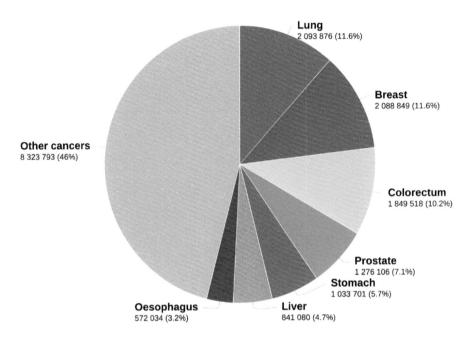

Total: 18,078,957

Fig. 2. Estimated number of new cases in 2018, worldwide, both sexes, all ages. (Data source: Globocan 2018 Graph production: Global Cancer Observatory (http://gco.iarc.fr).)

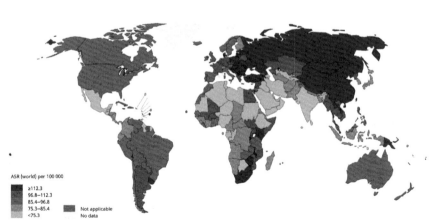

Fig. 3. Estimated age-standardized mortality rates (world) in 2018, all cancers, both sexes, all ages. All rights reserved. The designations used and the presentation of the material in this publication do not imply the expression of any opinion whatsoever on the part of the World Health Organization/IARC concerning the legal status of any country, territory, city, or area or of its authorities or concerning the delimitation of its frontiers or boundaries. Dotted and dashed lines on maps represent approximate borderlines for which there may not yet be full agreement. (Data source: GLOBOCAN 2018 Graph production: IARC (http://gco.iarc.fr/today) World Health Organization.)

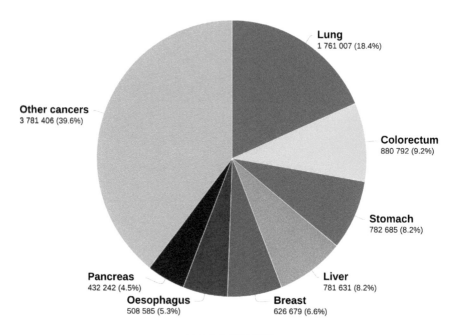

Fig. 4. Estimated number of deaths in 2018, worldwide, both sexes, all ages. (Data source: Globocan 2018 Graph production: Global Cancer Observatory (http://gco.iarc.fr).))

annually, and in situ cancers (except urinary bladder) of the breast (n = 48,530) and melanoma (n = 95,710).[8] The estimated number of new cases in 2020 for the 4 major cancers by sex and age group is shown in **Table 1**. Overall, death from cancer is the second leading cause of death in the United States behind heart disease, but by 2002, cancer was the leading cause of death in adults younger than age 85, which make up 98% of the population.[9] By 2020, the greater decline in death from heart disease is projected to lead to cancer being the leading cause of death in the United States.[10] Cancer also is the leading cause of premature mortality in the United States, that is, a measure estimated by applying life table data to each death from cancer based on remaining years of life left for an average person of the same sex, age, and race,[11] accounting for 9.3 million person-years of life lost (PYLL) in 2017, compared with 7.8 million PYLL for heart disease, and an average of 15.5 years of potential life lost (YPLL) due to death from cancer compared with 12.0 YPLL attributable to a death from heart disease.[11] The estimated number of deaths in 2020 for the 4 major cancers by sex and age group is shown in **Table 2**.

The cancer death rate has declined continuously since 1991, an overall decline of 29%, driven by long-term declines in death rates from lung, colorectal, breast, and prostate cancers that translates into 2.9 million fewer deaths than would have occurred if the peak rate in 1991 had remained the same.[7] In the United States, the top 3 causes of cancer deaths—lung and bronchus, prostate, and colon and rectum for men, and lung and bronchus, breast, and colon and rectum for women—42% and 45% of all cancer deaths, respectively, are cancers for which the efficacy of cancer screening has been established.[7]

Table 1
Estimated number of new cases for the 4 major cancers by sex and age group, 2020

	All Ages	Younger than 45	45 and Older	Younger than 65	65 and Older
All sites					
Male	893,660	54,090	839,570	372,260	521,400
Female	912,930	92,960	819,970	434,700	478,230
Colon and rectum					
Male	78,300	4830	73,470	37,990	40,310
Female	69,650	4730	64,920	29,950	39,700
Lung and bronchus					
Male	116,300	1190	115,110	35,680	80,620
Female	112,520	1400	111,120	34,570	77,950
Breast (female)	276,480	26,500	249,980	149,120	127,360
Prostate	191,930	760	191,170	77,000	114,930

Projected cases are based on incidence data during 2002 to 2016 from 49 states and the District of Columbia, as reported by the North American Association of Central Cancer Registries. Note: Estimates should not be compared with those from previous years.

From The American Cancer Society. Estimated New Cases for the Four Major Cancers by Sex & Age Group, 2020 (PDF). Available at: https://www.cancer.org/content/dam/cancer-org/research/cancer-facts-and-statistics/annual-cancer-facts-and-figures/2020/estimated-number-new-cases-by-sex-and-age-group-2020.pdf With permission.

Table 2
Estimated number of deaths for the 4 major cancers by sex and age group, 2020

	All Ages	Younger than 45	45 and Older	Younger than 65	65 and Older
All sites					
Male	321,160	8160	313,000	92,300	228,860
Female	285,360	9340	276,020	83,150	202,210
Colon and rectum					
Male	28,630	1010	27,620	10,100	18,530
Female	24,570	820	23,750	6920	17,650
Lung and bronchus					
Male	72,500	510	71,990	19,410	53,090
Female	63,220	420	62,800	15,930	47,290
Breast (female)	42,170	2320	39,850	16,350	25,820
Prostate	33,330	[a]	[a]	3540	29,790

Projected deaths are based on US mortality data from 2003 to 2017 as reported by the National Center for Health Statistics, Centers for Disease Control and Prevention. Note: Estimates should not be compared with those from previous years.

[a] Estimate for men less than age 45 y is fewer than 50 deaths.

From The American Cancer Society. Estimated Deaths for the Four Major Cancers by Sex & Age Group, 2020 (PDF). Available at: https://www.cancer.org/content/dam/cancer-org/research/cancer-facts-and-statistics/annual-cancer-facts-and-figures/2020/estimated-number-deaths-by-sex-and-age-group-2020.pdf With Permission.

Table 3
Five-year relative survival rates[a] (%) by stage at diagnosis, 2009–2015

	All Stages	Local	Regional	Distant		All Stages	Local	Regional	Distant
Breast (female)	90	99	86	27	Oral cavity and pharynx	65	84	66	39
Colon and rectum	64	90	71	14	Ovary	48	92	75	29
Colon	63	90	71	14	Pancreas	9	37	12	3
Rectum	67	89	71	15	Prostate	98	>99	>99	31
Esophagus	20	47	25	5	Stomach	32	69	31	5
Kidney[b]	75	93	70	12	Testis	95	99	96	73
Larynx	60	77	45	33	Thyroid	98	>99	98	56
Liver[c]	18	33	11	2	Urinary bladder[d]	77	70	36	5
Lung and bronchus	19	57	31	5	Uterine cervix	66	92	56	17
Melanoma of the skin	92	99	65	25	Uterine corpus	81	95	69	17

Local: an invasive malignant cancer confined entirely to the organ of origin. Regional: a malignant cancer that (1) has extended beyond the limits of the organ of origin directly into surrounding organs or tissues; (2) involves regional lymph nodes; or (3) has both regional extension and involvement of regional lymph nodes. Distant: a malignant cancer that has spread to parts of the body remote from the primary tumor either by direct extension or by discontinuous metastasis to distant organs, tissues, or via the lymphatic system to distant lymph nodes.
[a] Rates are adjusted for normal life expectancy and are based on cases diagnosed in the SEER 18 areas from 2009 to 2015, all followed through 2016.
[b] Includes renal pelvis.
[c] Includes intrahepatic bile duct.
[d] Rate for in situ cases is 96%.
Adapted from Howlader N, Noone AM, Krapcho M, Miller D, Brest A, Yu M, Ruhl J, Tatalovich Z, Mariotto A, Lewis DR, Chen HS, Feuer EJ, Cronin KA (eds). SEER Cancer Statistics Review, 1975-2016, National Cancer Institute. Bethesda, MD, https://seer.cancer.gov/csr/1975_2016/, based on November 2018 SEER data submission, posted to the SEER web site, April 2019.

THE ROLE OF PREVENTION AND EARLY DETECTION IN THE CONTROL OF CANCER

The control of cancer is and will continue to be a formidable challenge, although contributions from the accumulation of knowledge about disease etiology and natural history, opportunities for prevention and early detection, and advances in therapy have contributed to a reduction in the burden of disease over the past several decades. Among these strategies, few would disagree that preventing the occurrence of cancer is most desirable. The best example of a long-standing prevention-related cancer control strategy has been tobacco control—various strategies to prevent the uptake of cigarette smoking and to assist people who smoke to quit.[12] Other strategies exist, such as vaccinating children with against infection with human papillomavirus (HPV) to prevent HPV-related cancers[13,14] and the interrelationship of the contributions of obesity, sedentary lifestyle, unhealthy diet, and alcohol to the incidence of cancer and cancer outcomes.[15–17] Following cancer prevention guidelines also has been shown to reduce risk of other leading chronic conditions, given that the major causes of premature death in the United States share common risk factors.[18] According to American Cancer Society (ACS) researchers, at least 42% of the estimated new cancers in 2020 potentially were preventable, including 19% of all cancers that are attributable to smoking and 18% attributable to excess body weight, alcohol consumption, poor nutrition, and physical inactivity.[8] Cancers attributable to infectious agents, that is, HPV, hepatitis B virus, hepatitis C virus, and *Helicobacter pylori*, potentially are preventable through vaccination, behavioral change, or treatment of active infections.[19] Cancer prevention strategies at the individual and population levels are long-term investment strategies, for which reductions in cancer incidence and mortality will be reaped through adherence to recommendations and continuous efforts to promote risk reduction. As discussed previously, most of the preventive health objectives also are associated with a reduction in risk of cardiovascular disease, diabetes, and other chronic conditions and thus are worthy of persistent promotion in the primary care setting.[20]

Preventive strategies do not exist for all cancers nor are they certain to prevent the cancers for which risk reduction has been associated with protective behaviors. Protective behaviors are associated with a reduction in risk and thus are worthy for individuals to adopt, but they are not a guarantee against developing cancer. Furthermore, cancer prevention no longer is an option for the several millions of individuals who are diagnosed each year with invasive and in situ cancers of the body and skin, nor is it an option for the many more millions of individuals who presently have occult, undiagnosed disease that eventually will produce symptoms if not detected early. For these individuals, the control of cancer and the possibility of avoiding a premature death are dependent on successful treatment. Yet, survival statistics provide a stark reminder that treatment does not always assure the cure of disease, especially with cancer diagnosed at an advanced stage (**Table 3**).[7] Thus, the potential to prevent adverse cancer outcomes must be viewed as a combined commitment to prevention and early detection, with the latter achieved through adherence with recommended screening guidelines as well as being responsive to symptoms associated with cancer.

Cancer screening and early detection are associated with significantly better outcomes in breast, cervical, colorectal, lung, and prostate cancers, where first-generation prognostic factors (tumor size and grade, nodal invasion, and the presence of distant metastasis) still are the primary determinants of prognosis, and prognosis generally is better and treatment more successful if the disease is detected while still localized (see **Table 3**).[21] Approximately half of the expected new cases diagnosed each year are among cancers for which early cancer detection recommendations exist.[21]

THE ROLE OF CANCER SCREENING IN THE CONTROL OF CANCER

Cancer screening is a form of secondary prevention, that is, "the application of various tests to apparently healthy individuals to sort out those who probably have risk factors or are in the early stages of specified conditions."[22] Secondary prevention of cancer is equally essential as primary prevention in an individual's preventive health plan, and focuses on (1) detecting and treating early invasive disease and thus reducing the morbidity and risk of mortality associated with a diagnosis of advanced disease and (2) detecting precursor lesions known to be potentially precancerous and predictive of eventual malignancy, and by treating them, preventing progression to invasive disease. Detection of precancerous lesions of the cervix and colorectal adenomas are the 2 principle examples. Screening for cancer is a secondary prevention strategy.

In the United States, cancer screening is not organized; rather, it is opportunistic. Most cancer screening in industrialized countries is organized, that is, invitations to screening are sent to the target population from a centralized authority. Higher rates of attendance are possible because invitations are sent routinely when screening is due and result in direct outreach to the entire eligible population. If a patient needs follow-up care, such as additional imaging or biopsy, this also is tracked using the same centralized system and thus can be monitored for completion of the follow-up examination or test. An organized program also commonly includes monitoring of quality assurance issues, and ongoing evaluation of the program's performance. In contrast, in the United States, most cancer screening occurs as a coincidence of opportunity and interest during patient encounters for acute or chronic care or during a preventive health checkup. Without an encounter, an adult may be notified that a screening examination is due, but this notification is not assured, varies across health systems, and varies by the screening tests that an individual should receive. Thus, a 55-year -old woman may be able to depend on receiving a notification that she is due for her mammogram but likely will not receive any outreach for cervical cancer screening or colorectal cancer screening and depend on her primary care physician to remind her when these screening tests are due. If she does not have an encounter with her primary care physician, she may fail to be adherent with recommended screening intervals.

In the primary care setting, successful cancer screening is enhanced measurably by implementing the features of an organized system and, as much as possible, practicing population-based medicine. Two key elements to successful cancer screening in the primary care setting are risk assessment and the utilization of office tools for reminders and tracking cancer screening.

Risk Assessment

Although most adults are within a range of absolute risk that can be judged to be average, some adults would be judged to be at higher risk due to an inherited or acquired predisposition to cancer. For example, adults with a family history of cancer are at higher risk for the same cancer, in some instances, other cancers as well, and, depending on the pattern of family history, may be at higher risk for a diagnosis at an earlier age than when screening is recommended to begin in average risk adults. If a family history suggests a patient may be carrying a deleterious mutation on a cancer susceptibility gene, then referral to genetic counseling and testing may be warranted. For these reasons, a family history of cancer on both the maternal and paternal side extending at least to 2 generations that includes the type of cancer and age at diagnosis must be collected no later than the age at which early screening would begin if the patient was determined to be at inherited risk. There is an extensive literature, however, on the failure in primary care to take a thorough family history, update it periodically, and act on the information that was gathered.[23–26] Numerous tools exist for taking family history,[27] and there is clear evidence that patients report family histories accurately and are able to complete family histories at home or online, which results in time savings.[28,29] The Centers for Disease Control and Prevention have extensive family health history resources that are evidence based and can be implemented into the primary care practice.[30]

Reminder Systems

Historically, the most common explanation patients have given for why they had a screening test is that their doctor advised them to get one, and, likewise, the most common explanation for not having had a screening test is their doctor did not advise them to get one. In the absence of an organized system that sends invitations to adults when they are due for cancer screening, the inefficiency of encounters with health services to provide a referral is relied on. These encounters may not occur, however, coincident with when cancer screening is due, there may not be time to address cancer screening during a visit for acute or chronic care, and the need for cancer screening simply may be overlooked. Reminder systems of every kind, from notes in a patient's chart to electronic systems and patient outreach by phone or mail, have been shown to be effective in increasing cancer screening rates.[31] Moreover, the practice should regularly utilize the electronic health record to assess the proportion of patients who are adherent with cancer screening recommendations, remind those who are due for cancer screening and provide referrals, and monitor their adherence to the reminder for screening.

UTILIZATION OF CANCER SCREENING IN THE UNITED STATES

The most recent data from the 2015 National Health Interview Study (NHIS) show that breast cancer screening rates have changed little from 2005 to 2015 (**Table 4**).[32] Approximately only half of women ages 40+ report a mammogram in the past year, and, although a higher percentage of women report having had a mammogram in the past 2 years, these data cannot be interpreted as reflecting adherence to annual versus biennial screening. **Table 5** shows reported mammography screening rates in 2015 by education, race/ethnicity, and health insurance status among adults less than age 64.[32] There is a clear, linear association between education and reporting a recent mammogram, but the greater disparity is seen among women who report that they do not have health insurance.

As seen in **Table 4**, NHIS colorectal cancer screening rates have increased from 46.8% in 2005% to 62.6% in 2015. Although colorectal cancer screening rates have been rising, screening in adults aged 50 to 54 lags well behind screening in those over age 60, a clear indication that uptake of colorectal cancer screening is not being initiated at the age of 50 when most guidelines still recommend that screening should begin (the ACS recommends beginning colorectal cancer screening at age 45[33]). In the 2015 NHIS data, only 48% of people aged 50 to 54 years report being up to date with screening.[32] One factor that has been shown to limit uptake of colorectal cancer screening is referral only to colonoscopy, rather than giving patients a choice between an invasive test or a noninvasive tests, such as a high-sensitivity stool test.[34] In a randomized trial examining the uptake of screening among adults who were

Table 4
Colorectal, breast, cervical, prostate, and lung cancer screening prevalence, National Health Interview Survey 2005–2015[b]

	2005 (%)	2008 (%)	2010 (%)	2013 (%)	2015 (%)	Absolute Change (2015–2005) (%)
Colorectal cancer (adults aged ≥50 y)						
Up-to-date[c]	46.8	53.2	59.1	58.6	62.6	15.8
Up-to-date (including CT colonography)[d]	—	—	59.2	—	62.6	
Colonoscopy in the past 10 y	39.2	48.0	55.5	55.2	59.8	20.6
Sigmoidoscopy in the past 5 y	3.9	2.2	3.5	3.6	2.5	−1.5
Stool-based testing in the past year[e]	12.1	10.0	8.8	7.8	7.2	−4.9
CT Colonography in the past 5 y	—	—	<1.0[a]	—	<1.0[a]	—
Colorectal cancer (adults aged ≥45 y)						
Up-to-date[c]	40.7	44.7	51.9	51.9	55.4	14.7
Up-to-date (including CT colonography)[d]	—	—	52.0	—	55.5	
Colonoscopy in the past 10 y	34.1	42.0	48.6	48.7	52.9	18.8
Sigmoidoscopy in the past 5 y	3.3	1.9	3.1	3.3	2.2	−1.1
Stool-based testing in the past year[e]	10.5	8.7	7.6	6.8	6.3	−4.2
CT Colonography in the past 5 y			<1.0[a]		<1.0[a]	
Breast cancer (women aged ≥40 y)						
Mammogram in the past year	51.2	53	50.8	51.3	50.2	−1.0
Breast cancer (women aged 40–54 y)						
Mammogram in the past year	49.3	49.4	48.8	50.0	48.4	−0.9
Breast cancer screening (women ≥55 y)						
Mammogram in the past year	54.1	57.9	54.2	53.9	53.1	−1.0
Mammogram in the past 2 y	69.0	71.5	69.1	69.4	67.7	−1.3
Cervical cancer (women 21–65 y)						
Pap test in the past 3 y[f]	85.4	84.6	83.1	80.9	81.6	−3.8
Prostate cancer (men aged ≥50 y)						
PSA test in the past year[g]	40.7	44.1	41.3	34.5	34.4	−6.3
Lung cancer among high-risk smokers (55–80 y)[h]						
LDCT in the past year	—	—	3.3	—	3.9	—

Abbreviations: CRC, colorectal cancer cancer; CT, computed tomography; y, years.

[a] Relative standard error exceeds 30%, unstable estimate. Estimated prevalence was less than 1%.

[b] Estimates for colorectal, breast, cervical, and prostate cancer screening are age-adjusted to the 2000 US standard population.

[c] Up-to-date CRC screening included stool-based tests within the preceding year, or sigmoidoscopy within the preceding 5 y, or colonoscopy within the preceding 10 y.

[d] Up-to-date CRC screening included stool-based tests within the preceding year, or sigmoidoscopy within the preceding 5 y, or colonoscopy within the preceding 10 y, or CT colonography in the past 5 y. Data on CT colonography were collected only in 2010 and 2015.

[e] Stool-based tests included fecal occult blood tests or fecal immunochemical tests using a home test kit.

[f] Pap testing was measured among women with intact uteri.

[g] Among men without a history of prostate cancer.

[h] Among high-risk smokers defined as people ages 55 y to 80 y who have ≥30 pack-year smoking history and currently smoke or have quit within the past 15 y.

From Wender RC, Brawley OW, Fedewa SA, Gansler T, Smith RA. A blueprint for cancer screening and early detection: Advancing screening's contribution to cancer control. CA Cancer J Clin. 2019;69(1):50-79; with permission.

Table 5

Colorectal, breast, cervical, prostate, and lung cancer screening prevalence according to race/ethnicity, insurance, and educational attainment, National Health Interview Survey, 2015[c]

	Hispanic (%)	Race and Ethnicity			Health Insurance (<64 Years of Age)		Educational Level			
		White, Non-Hispanic (%)	Black, Non-Hispanic (%)	Asian (%)	Yes (%)	No (%)	Some High School or Less (%)	High School Diploma or General Equivalency Diploma (%)	Some College (%)	College Graduate (%)
Colorectal cancer (adults aged ≥50 y)										
Up-to-date[d]	49.9	65.4	61.8	49.4	59.6	25.1	47.4	58.6	64.3	71.3
Up-to-date (including CT colonography)[e]	50.0	65.5	61.8	49.1	59.6	25.1	47.4	58.5	64.4	71.3
Colonoscopy in the past 10 y	46.8	63.0	58.3	44.3	56.4	23.5	44.7	56.1	61.3	68.4
Sigmoidoscopy in the past 5 y	3.3	2.4	2.5	2.0	1.9	<1.0[a]	2.8	1.8	2.4	3.0
Stool-based testing in the past year[f]	7.3	6.9	8.0	9.2	6.2	4.0	6.3	7.1	7.2	7.7
CT Colonography in the past 5 y	<1.0[a]	<1.0[a]	<1.0[a]	<1.0[a]	<1.0[a]	<1.0[a]	<1.0[a]	<1.0[a]	<1.0[a]	<1.0[a]
Colorectal cancer (adults aged ≥45 y)										
Up-to-date[d]	41.4	58.7	55.1	43.1	47.6	20.8	41.4	51.9	57.3	62.8
Up-to-date (including CT colonography)[e]	41.4	58.8	55.2	42.9	47.7	20.8	41.4	51.8	57.4	62.9
Colonoscopy in the past 10 y	38.6	56.4	51.8	38.6	45.1	19.4	38.8	49.6	54.5	60.2

(continued on next page)

Table 5
(continued)

	Race and Ethnicity				Health Insurance (<64 Years of Age)		Educational Level			
	Hispanic (%)	White, Non-Hispanic (%)	Black, Non-Hispanic (%)	Asian (%)	Yes (%)	No (%)	Some High School or Less (%)	High School Diploma or General Equivalency Diploma (%)	Some College (%)	College Graduate (%)
Sigmoidoscopy in the past 5 y	2.9	2.1	2.2	1.8	1.6	<1.0[a]	2.5	1.5	2.1	2.5
Stool-based testing in the past year[f]	6.1	6.1	7.1	7.7	4.8	3.2	5.5	6.2	6.3	6.8
CT colonography in the past 5 y[g]	<1.0[a]	<1.0[a]	<1.0[a]	<1.0[a]	<1.0[a]	<1.0[a]	<1.0[a]	<1.0[a]	<1.0[a]	<1.0[a]
Breast cancer (women aged ≥40 y)										
Mammogram in the past year	45.7	50.3	55.4	47.1	52.5	20.9	38.9	45.0	51.2	57.9
Breast cancer (women aged 40–54 y)										
Mammogram in the past year	43.7	48.3	55.2	49.8	51.6	20.3	39.9	41.3	50.0	53.8
Breast cancer screening (women ≥55 y)										
Mammogram in the past year	49.0	53.5	56.5	47.0	57.4	20.3	39.5	50.4	53.7	62.0
Mammogram in the past 2 y	65.4	68.0	70.9	60.1	74.1	31.4	51.9	64.7	67.8	78.1

Cervical cancer (women 21–65 y)										
Pap test in the past 3 y[h]	77.4	83.1	84.7	73.3	84.4	60.8	69.9	75.1	83.9	88.6
Prostate cancer (men aged ≥50 y)										
PSA test in the past year[i]	25.5	37.1	30.7	17.4	29.8	10.2	20.1	30.4	34.6	44.0
Lung cancer among high-risk smokers (55–80 y)[j]										
LDCT in the past year	<5.0[b]	4.1	<5.0[b]	<5.0[b]	<5.0[b]	<5.0[b]	<5.0[b]	<5.0[b]	<5.0[b]	<5.0[b]

Abbreviations: CRC, colorectal cancer cancer; CT, computed tomography.

[a] Relative standard error exceeds 30%, unstable estimate. Estimated prevalence was <1%.

[b] Relative standard error exceeds 30%, unstable estimate. Estimated prevalence was ≤5%.

[c] Estimates for colorectal, breast, cervical, and prostate cancer screening are age-adjusted to the 2000 US standard population.

[d] Up-to-date CRC screening included stool-based tests within the preceding year, or sigmoidoscopy within the preceding 5 y, or colonoscopy within the preceding 10 y.

[e] Up-to-date CRC screening included stool-based tests within the preceding year, or sigmoidoscopy within the preceding 5 y, or colonoscopy within the preceding 10 y, or CT colonography in the past 5 y. Data on CT colonography were only collected in 2010 and 2015.

[f] Stool-based tests included fecal occult blood tests or fecal immunochemical tests using a home test kit.

[g] Estimates for CT colonography are unstable, relative standard errors exceed 30%.

[h] Pap testing was measured among women with intact uteri.

[i] Among men without a history of prostate cancer.

[j] Among high risk smokers defined as people ages 55 y to 80 y who have ≥30 pack-year smoking history and currently smoke or have quit within the past 15 y. Estimates for LDCT according to sociodemographics are unstable.

From Wender RC, Brawley OW, Fedewa SA, Gansler T, Smith RA. A blueprint for cancer screening and early detection: Advancing screening's contribution to cancer control. CA Cancer J Clin. 2019;69(1):50-79; with permission.

offered only colonoscopy or a stool test, or both, significantly lower completion rates were observed among adults who were recommended to undergo colonoscopy (38%) compared with adults recommended to undergo fecal occult blood test (67%) or given a choice of either test (69%).[34] **Table 5** shows reported colorectal cancer screening rates in 2015 by race/ethnicity, health insurance among adults less than age 64, and education.[32]

The most recent data from the NHIS show that rates of cervical cancer screening with cytology every 3 years have declined from 85.4% in 2005 to 81.6% in 2015 (see **Table 4**).[32] **Table 5** shows reported cervical cancer screening rates in 2015 by race/ethnicity, health insurance among adults less than age 64, and education. Similar patterns are evident by educational attainment that are observed with other screening tests, but more than half of women without health insurance report that they recently have been screened for cervical cancer. The higher screening rate in uninsured women likely is attributable to the wide availability of cervical cancer screening programs for low-income women.

In 2005, NHIS data showed that 41% of men aged 50 years and older reported having undergone a prostate-specific antigen (PSA) test for prostate cancer screening in the previous year. Reported screening in the past year was highest in 2008 (44%) but declined to 35% in 2013 and has remained relatively stable since then (see **Table 4**).[32] The recent decline in PSA testing has been attributed to the change in the US Preventive Services Task Force (USPSTF) prostate cancer screening recommendation in 2012 from a recommendation for shared decision making (a C rating) to a recommendation against screening (a D rating),[35] which then was returned to a recommendation for shared decision making in the 2018 update.[36] In 2015, 63% of men 50 years and older reported receiving at least 1 element of shared decision making; only 17% of men with a recent PSA test reported participating in full shared decision making.[37]

Although lung cancer screening with low-dose computed tomography (LDCT) was not recommended until 2013[38,39] or covered by health plans and Medicare until 2015, the NHIS began collecting data on lung cancer screening in 2010. In 2010, only 3.3% of adults who meet USPSTF criteria (current or former smokers [quit <15 years] ages 55 years to 80 years with at least a 30 pack-year history) reported having had an LDCT for lung cancer screening in the past year, and, in 2015, this proportion was similar, at 3.9% (see **Table 4**).[32] **Table 5** shows reported lung cancer screening rates in 2015 by race/ethnicity, health insurance among adults less than age 64, and education.[40] It does appear from more recent survey data from the Centers for Disease Control and Prevention Behavioral Risk Factor Surveillance System survey conducted in 2017 in 10 states that rates of LDCT screening are increasing in the United States.[41] Among surveyed adults who met USPSTF eligibility criteria for LDCT screening, 12.5% reported having had an LDCT for lung cancer screening in the past year.[41]

SUMMARY

Beginning with cervical cancer screening in the 1950s, primary care clinicians have been called on to refer their patients to cancer screening for the past 70 years. Additional screening tests were introduced over this period—lung cancer screening with chest radiograph and colorectal cancer screening in the 1970s, breast cancer screening in the 1980s, and prostate cancer screening in the 1990s—and, many years after the efficacy of chest radiograph screening could not be demonstrated, LDCT screening for lung cancer is recommended again. Yet, the fullest potential of early cancer detection is not being met, even though it is within reach by simply applying the evidence hand and ensuring access to care to all Americans.[42] Put simply, the potential of cancer screening remains unfulfilled in the United States, because screening is poorly integrated into routine health care, there are enduring inequalities in access to care, and there is uneven quality in the delivery of cancer screening services. Screening under opportunistic conditions rather than through a system is inefficient at both the individual level and population levels[43]; moreover, without a system, there is no readiness to implement any new early detection technology that could improve health outcomes, as seen by the chronically low screening rates for lung cancer 6 years after it was given a B rating by the USPSTF. A comprehensive system of early detection potentially not only leads to high levels of participation but also ensures that all the elements of a program of early detection and intervention are highly competent, interrelated, and interdependent. A system has the potential not only to increase quality but also to reduce the volume of small errors that contribute to incremental erosion of efficiency as well as the volume of gross failures to prevent a death from cancer that was avoidable. Although there are many practical barriers that must be overcome to establish true population-based screening programs, a system of organized screening, overall, in a local health system, or even at the practice level holds the greatest potential to realize the benefits of reducing the incidence rate of advanced cancers and subsequently avoiding premature mortality.

In the near term, the greatest potential for reducing death from cancer is through early detection and appropriate treatment. Although some investigators have questioned the continued relevance of cancer screening in an era of improvements in cancer therapy,[44] no therapeutic agent exists that can match the prognostic advantage of being diagnosed with a localized cancer, let alone offer the advantage of preventing cancer by detecting and treating precursor lesions. In a recent study of the influence of attending mammography screening on the incidence rate of fatal breast cancer at 10 years and 20 years after diagnosis, the investigators observed substantially lower rates of fatal breast cancer of 60% and 47%, respectively, compared with women who did not attend screening.[45] This novel methodology measures the independent influence of attending screening because the 10-year and 20-year incidence rates of fatal breast cancer are based on year of diagnosis, when each women diagnosed with breast cancer would have received the state-of-the-art therapy for her stage at diagnosis. For any cancer for which screening is recommended, most adults who are diagnosed with cancer have better outcomes if they attended screening compared with those who did not.

The effectiveness cancer screening is dependent on the attendance rate, the sensitivity of the protocol, the management of positive findings, and timely access to treatment. The interrelatedness of these priorities is self-evident—achieving them routinely benefits from an organized care-delivery system, within which each of the key steps that need to occur is governed by rules, roles, relationships, and oversight.

Cancer screening in the primary care setting benefits from teamwork, an office policy, and a system to track risk, screening rates, and reminders. High-quality screening requires high rates of (1) standardized, timely, and routine risk assessment in order to identify and properly triage patients at high risk; (2) efficient, competent discussions with patients about what to expect from screening; (3) reminder and outreach systems to ensure patients receive regular screening at recommended intervals; (4) tracking patients with positive findings to ensure timely work-up of positive findings, diagnostic evaluation, and referral to treatment with minimal delay; and (5) awareness of the quality of the services where patients are being referred. Tools exist to support primary care providers to build a system to support their own patient panel[46]; additional resources are shown in **Box 1**.

Box 1
Useful online resources related to cancer screening

Cancer screening guidelines
ACS
The ACS has been publishing cancer screening guidelines since 1980. Current guidelines can be found on the ACS Web site, along with materials for patients. Previous guidelines are open access at *CA: A Cancer Journal for Clinicians.* The ACS publishes an annual review of its guidelines and current issues in cancer screening in *CA.* https://acsjournals.onlinelibrary.wiley.com/journal/15424863
https://www.cancer.org/healthy/find-cancer-early/cancer-screening-guidelines/american-cancer-society-guidelines-for-the-early-detection-of-cancer.html
USPSTF
The USPSTF has been publishing cancer screening recommendations as well as recommendations related to other clinical preventive services, such as screenings, counseling services, and preventive medications, since 1986. All recommendations as well as supporting systematic reviews and materials for patients are published on the USPSTF Web site and/or in a peer-reviewed journal.
https://uspreventiveservicestaskforce.org/uspstf/
National Comprehensive Cancer Network
The National Comprehensive Cancer Network was established in 1995 to develop and communicate scientific, evidence related to the detection and treatment of cancer to better inform the decision-making process between patients and physicians. Materials are available for clinicians and patients. https://www.nccn.org/professionals/physician_gls/default.aspx
ECRI Guidelines Trust
Founded as the Emergency Care Research Institute in 1968, ECRI is an organization dedicated to efficacy and cost-effectiveness of health care. The ECRI Guidelines Trust is a publicly available repository of clinical guidelines that was developed in 2018 in response to the defunding of the National Guideline Clearinghouse by the federal government.
https://guidelines.ecri.org/
Guideline sInternational Network
Guidelines International Network is an international network of guideline development organizations, implementers, researchers, students, and other stakeholders focused on leading, strengthening, and supporting collaboration and work within the guideline development, adaptation, and implementation community.
https://g-i-n.net/about-g-i-n/introduction

Guideline development and evaluation tools
Appraisal of Guidelines for Research and Evaluation
The Appraisal of Guidelines for Research and Evaluation (AGREE) instrument evaluates the process of practice guideline development and the quality of reporting. The AGREE II tool comprises 23 items organized into the original 6 quality domains.
https://www.agreetrust.org/
http://www.agreetrust.org/resource-centre/agree-reporting-checklist/
Grading of Recommendations Assessment, Development and Evaluation
The Grading of Recommendations Assessment, Development and Evaluation (GRADE) working group began in the year 2000 as an informal collaboration of people with an interest in addressing the shortcomings of grading systems in health care. The working group has developed a common, sensible, and transparent approach to grading quality (or certainty) of evidence and strength of recommendations. GRADE is the most widely used methodology for grading evidence and recommendations.
https://www.gradeworkinggroup.org/

Cancer statistics
ACS Facts and Figures
The ACS publishes an annual update on US cancer statistics, including state-level data on the leading cancers. An annual open-access article also is published in *CA: A Cancer Journal for Clinicians.* The Facts and Figures web site also includes regularly updated disease-specific reports on breast cancer and colorectal cancer and cancer prevention and early detection and an interactive tool for producing tailored cancer statistics charts and graphs.

https://www.cancer.org/research/cancer-facts-statistics/all-cancer-facts-figures/cancer-facts-figures-2020.html

Centers for Disease Control and Prevention
The Centers for Disease Control and Prevention is a source for national, state, and county data on cancer as well as state profiles that include disease burden and screening rates.
https://www.cdc.gov/cancer/dcpc/data/index.htm
https://www.statecancerprofiles.cancer.gov/index.html

National Cancer Institute Surveillance, Epidemiology, and End Results program
The Surveillance, Epidemiology, and End Results (SEER) program provides information on cancer statistics in an effort to reduce the cancer burden among the US population. SEER is supported by the Surveillance Research Program in the National Cancer Institute Division of Cancer Control and Population Sciences. The SEER Web site has an interactive analytical tool as well as access to the annual Cancer Statistics Review, a report of the most recent cancer incidence, mortality, survival, prevalence, and lifetime risk statistics for the United States.
https://seer.cancer.gov/

IARC Global Cancer Observatory
The Global Cancer Observatory is an interactive Web-based platform presenting global cancer statistics to inform cancer control and research.
https://gco.iarc.fr/

Cancer screening is widely accepted by the population but often controversial and regularly scrutinized for the benefit-to-harm ratio, for which there are no benchmarks or thresholds for acceptable versus unacceptable rates. Ideally, a system could lead to improvements in benefits and a reduction in spectrum of occurrences that fall into the category of harms. In 2003, Peter Sasieni[47] pointed out that citing the number needed to screen to prevent one death, and making a judgment about that number, equated screening with treatment, to which he added, "it is not treatment." Instead, he added, screening should be thought about as insurance. He added further, "Insurance is put in place to avoid catastrophic consequences of an unlikely event."[47] Most people will not develop cancer in their lifetime. They should be aware not only of the common negative experiences of cancer screening but also the very serious, potentially life-changing and life-taking consequences of being diagnosed with an advanced-stage cancer. Primary care clinicians should adopt this line of thinking for themselves and their patients and advocate for the systems and payment reform that will make it easier for them to fully integrate a system of cancer screening into their practice.

DISCLOSURE

The authors have nothing to disclose.

REFERENCES

1. International Agency for Research on Cancer. Launch of IARC Cancer Screening in Five Continents (CanScreen5) website. Available at: https://www.iarc.fr/news-events/launch_canscreen5/. Accessed July 22, 2020.

2. Murillo R. Screening: From Biology to Public Health. In: Wild CP, Weiderpass E, Stewart BW, editors. World cancer report: cancer research for cancer prevention. Lyon (France): International Agency for Research on Cancer; 2020. p. 540–9.

3. International Agency for Research on Cancer. All Cancers–Source: Globocan 2018. Available at: https://gco.iarc.fr/today/data/factsheets/cancers/39-All-cancers-fact-sheet.pdf. Accessed July 22, 2020.

4. International Agency for Research on Cancer. Cancer Tomorrow. Available at: https://gco.iarc.fr/tomorrow/home. Accessed July 22, 2020.
5. Cao B, Soejomataram I, Bray F. The burden and prevention of premature deaths from noncommunicable diseases, including cancer: a global perspective. In: Wild CP, Weiderpass E, Stewart BW, editors. World cancer report: cancer research for cancer prevention. Lyon (France): International Agency for Research on Cancer; 2020. p. 16–22.
6. Soejomataram I, Bray F. Global trends in cancer incidence and mortality. In: Wild CP, Weiderpass E, Stewart BW, editors. World cancer report: cancer research for cancer prevention. Lyon (France): International Agency for Research on Cancer; 2020. p. 23–33.
7. Siegel RL, Miller KD, Jemal A. Cancer statistics, 2020. CA Cancer J Clin 2020; 70:7–30.
8. American Cancer Society. American Cancer Society Facts and Figures 2020. Atlanta (GA): American Cancer Society; 2020.
9. Jemal A, Murray T, Ward E, et al. Cancer statistics, 2005. CA Cancer J Clin 2005; 55:10–30.
10. Weir HK, Anderson RN, Coleman King SM, et al. Heart disease and cancer deaths - trends and projections in the United States, 1969-2020. Prev Chronic Dis 2016;13:E157.
11. Howlader N, Noone AM, Krapcho M, et al. SEER ancer statistics review, 1975-2017. Bethesda (MD): National Cancer Institute; 2020.
12. Kathuria H, Neptune E. Primary and secondary prevention of lung cancer: tobacco treatment. Clin Chest Med 2020;41:39–51.
13. Senkomago V, Henley SJ, Thomas CC, et al. Human papillomavirus-attributable cancers - United States, 2012-2016. MMWR Morb Mortal Wkly Rep 2019;68: 724–8.
14. Saslow D, Andrews KS, Manassaram-Baptiste D, et al, American Cancer Society Guideline Development Group. Human papillomavirus vaccination 2020 guideline update: American Cancer Society guideline adaptation. CA Cancer J Clin 2020;70(4):274–80.
15. Rock CL, Thomson C, Gansler T, et al. American Cancer Society guideline for diet and physical activity for cancer prevention. CA Cancer J Clin 2020;70(4):245–71.
16. Emmons KM, Colditz GA. Realizing the potential of cancer prevention - the role of implementation science. N Engl J Med 2017;376:986–90.
17. Colditz GA, Emmons KM. Accelerating the pace of cancer prevention- right now. Cancer Prev Res (Phila) 2018;11:171–84.
18. McCullough ML, Patel AV, Kushi LH, et al. Following cancer prevention guidelines reduces risk of cancer, cardiovascular disease, and all-cause mortality. Cancer Epidemiol Biomarkers Prev 2011;20:1089–97.
19. de Martel C, Franceschi S. Infections and cancer: established associations and new hypotheses. Crit Rev Oncol Hematol 2009;70:183–94.
20. Kahn R, Robertson RM, Smith R, et al. The impact of prevention on reducing the burden of cardiovascular disease. Circulation 2008;118:576–85.
21. Smith RA, Andrews KS, Brooks D, et al. Cancer screening in the United States, 2019: A review of current American Cancer Society guidelines and current issues in cancer screening. CA Cancer J Clin 2019;69:184–210.
22. Morrison AS. Screening in chronic disease. New York: Oxford University Press; 1992.
23. Ginsburg GS, Wu RR, Orlando LA. Family health history: underused for actionable risk assessment. Lancet 2019;394:596–603.

24. Wood ME, Stockdale A, Flynn BS. Interviews with primary care physicians regarding taking and interpreting the cancer family history. Fam Pract 2008;25: 334–40.
25. Murff HJ, Greevy RA, Syngal S. The comprehensiveness of family cancer history assessments in primary care. Community Genet 2007;10:174–80.
26. Murff HJ, Spigel DR, Syngal S. Does this patient have a family history of cancer? An evidence-based analysis of the accuracy of family cancer history. JAMA 2004; 292:1480–9.
27. Cleophat JE, Nabi H, Pelletier S, et al. What characterizes cancer family history collection tools? A critical literature review. Curr Oncol 2018;25:e335–50.
28. Qureshi N, Carroll JC, Wilson B, et al. The current state of cancer family history collection tools in primary care: a systematic review. Genet Med 2009;11: 495–506.
29. Acheson LS, Zyzanski SJ, Stange KC, et al. Validation of a self-administered, computerized tool for collecting and displaying the family history of cancer. J Clin Oncol 2006;24:5395–402.
30. Centers for Disease Control and Prevention. Family Health History. Available at: https://www.cdc.gov/genomics/famhistory/index.htm. Accessed July 24, 2020.
31. Sabatino SA, Lawrence B, Elder R, et al. Effectiveness of interventions to increase screening for breast, cervical, and colorectal cancers: nine updated systematic reviews for the guide to community preventive services. Am J Prev Med 2012; 43:97–118.
32. National Center for Health Statistics. National Health Interview Survey. Available at: https://www.cdc.gov/nchs/nhis/about_nhis.htm. Accessed November 23, 2018.
33. Wolf AMD, Fontham ETH, Church TR, et al. Colorectal cancer screening for average-risk adults: 2018 guideline update from the American Cancer Society. CA Cancer J Clin 2018;68:250–81.
34. Inadomi JM, Vijan S, Janz NK, et al. Adherence to colorectal cancer screening: a randomized clinical trial of competing strategies. Arch Intern Med 2012;172: 575–82.
35. Jemal A, Fedewa SA, Ma J, et al. Prostate cancer incidence and PSA testing patterns in relation to USPSTF screening recommendations. JAMA 2015;314: 2054–61.
36. U. S. Preventive Services Task Force, Grossman DC, Curry SJ, et al. Screening for prostate cancer: US preventive services task force recommendation statement. JAMA 2018;319:1901–13.
37. Fedewa SA, Gansler T, Smith R, et al. Recent patterns in shared decision making for prostate-specific antigen testing in the United States. Ann Fam Med 2018;16: 139–44.
38. Wender R, Fontham ET, Barrera E Jr, et al. American Cancer Society lung cancer screening guidelines. CA Cancer J Clin 2013;63:107–17.
39. Moyer VA, Force USPST. Screening for lung cancer: U.S. Preventive Services Task Force recommendation statement. Ann Intern Med 2014;160:330–8.
40. Jemal A, Fedewa SA. Lung Cancer Screening With Low-Dose Computed Tomography in the United States-2010 to 2015. JAMA Oncol 2017;3:1278–81.
41. Richards TB, Soman A, Thomas CC, et al. Screening for lung cancer - 10 States, 2017. MMWR Morb Mortal Wkly Rep 2020;69:201–6.
42. Wender RC, Brawley OW, Fedewa SA, et al. A blueprint for cancer screening and early detection: Advancing screening's contribution to cancer control. CA Cancer J Clin 2019;69:50–79.

43. Miles A, Cockburn J, Smith RA, et al. A perspective from countries using organized screening programs. Cancer 2004;101:1201–13.
44. Welch HG. Screening mammography–a long run for a short slide? N Engl J Med 2010;363:1276–8.
45. Tabar L, Dean PB, Chen TH, et al. The incidence of fatal breast cancer measures the increased effectiveness of therapy in women participating in mammography screening. Cancer 2019;125:515–23.
46. National Colorectal Cancer Roundtable. National Colorectal Cancer Roundtable Website. Available at: http://nccrt.org. Accessed July 23, 2020.
47. Sasieni PD. Outcomes of screening to prevent cancer: think of screening as insurance. BMJ 2003;327:50 [author reply: 50].

The Evaluation of Cancer Screening

Concepts and Outcome Measures

Stephen W. Duffy, MSc[a],*, Robert A. Smith, PhD[b]

KEYWORDS

- Screening • Cancer • Evaluation • Methodology

KEY POINTS

- Cancer screening evaluation is a specialist area of healthcare evaluation, requiring specific skills and methods.
- Evaluation may have different purposes, including proof of principle, quality control of screening services, or assessment of innovative screening technology.
- Methods of evaluation will depend on both the purpose and the primary object of screening (prevention or early detection).

INTRODUCTION

Before considering evaluation of cancer screening, we should probably describe what cancer screening is, and before that we should define medical screening more generally. An eloquent and useful definition of screening has been given by Wald as "... the systematic application of a test or enquiry to identify individuals at sufficient risk of a specific disorder to warrant further investigation or direct preventive action, amongst persons who have not sought medical attention on account of symptoms of that disorder."[1]

The preceding definition is clearly very general and can cover a wide range of investigations, conditions, and mechanisms of action. However, one point on which it is very specific is the population to which the screening is applied: persons who have not sought medical attention on account of symptoms of that disorder. If a test is applied to persons who have sought medical advice for symptoms, this is not screening, it is diagnosis.

Cancer screening encompasses a wide range of investigations, aims, and mechanisms of achieving those aims. Major potential screening investigation strategies include:

[a] Wolfson Institute of Preventive Medicine, Queen Mary University of London, Charterhouse Square, London EC1M 6BQ, UK; [b] American Cancer Society, 250 Williams Street, Atlanta, GA 30303, USA
* Corresponding author.
E-mail address: s.w.duffy@qmul.ac.uk

Med Clin N Am 104 (2020) 939–953
https://doi.org/10.1016/j.mcna.2020.07.002
0025-7125/20/© 2020 Elsevier Inc. All rights reserved.

medical.theclinics.com

- Imaging: for example radiographic mammography for breast cancer, low-dose computed tomography for lung cancer.
- Examination of exfoliated cells: examples include cervical smears, now largely replaced or being replaced by human papillomavirus testing.
- Visual examination: examples include unassisted visual examination of the skin for atypical nevi or melanoma, and more invasive approaches including colonoscopy for colorectal cancer.
- Biomarkers: for example circulating markers of disease, such as prostate-specific antigen (PSA) for prostate cancer.
- Palpation: examples include clinical examination of the breasts, and digital rectal examination.

This list is by no means exhaustive, but gives an idea of the range of potential cancer screening tests. There is similarly a range of clinical aims and mechanisms. For instance, mammography screening for breast cancer is aimed at detecting breast cancer at an earlier stage when treatment is more likely to be successful, compared with when breast cancer is diagnosed symptomatically.[2] Colonoscopy and sigmoidoscopy, on the other hand, are aimed primarily at detecting precancerous adenomas, removing them, and thus preventing them from progressing to cancer at all.[3]

One further point to note with respect to cancer screening: in general, the screening test does not diagnose the cancer. It generally identifies those who need further investigation. To take the example of breast cancer screening, a positive screening mammogram is not a diagnosis of breast cancer. In the National Health Service Breast Screening Programme in the United Kingdom, on average, 1 in 5 women recalled for further investigation following a suspicious screening mammogram actually have breast cancer. The test is not expected to distinguish perfectly between those who do and do not have the disease, but the extent to which it does is an important ingredient in evaluation.

In this article, we review the main tools available for evaluation of cancer screening, in terms of the following:

1. Proof of principle: does the screening prevent mortality or significant morbidity from the cancer?
2. Service evaluation: is a routine service screening program (ie, screening in the community) delivering the expected clinical benefits?
3. Program quality: is a screening program meeting standards of test accuracy, punctuality, minimization of screening side effects, and so forth?
4. Innovation: should an existing screening program change to a new technology?

CANCER SCREENING EVALUATION TECHNIQUES: PROOF OF PRINCIPLE
Randomized Trials of Screening

Cancer screening as a public health activity is not a case-finding exercise. Its role is to prevent premature mortality or significant morbidity from the cancer in question. A major task of cancer research is to design studies that will inform policy makers as to whether it does so. Let us first take the case in which the screening aims to detect cancer, but at an early stage, when treatment is more likely to be successful in preventing death from the disease.

At this point, we briefly mention the 2 classic biases, *lead time bias* and *length bias*, which screening reviews perennially discuss, but which have been known about for decades.[4] With respect to lead time, if screening is successful in detecting cancer early, it necessarily confers an increase in the time from diagnosis to death, that is, an increase in survival time. This would occur whether or not the screening prevented or delayed death from the disease in question. Length bias refers to the phenomenon whereby comparison of outcomes between screen-detected and symptomatic cancers is biased by the fact that less aggressive tumors are likely to grow more slowly and therefore have a longer window of opportunity for screen detection.

It should be noted here that the preceding does not mean that lead time is a bad thing: for screening to be effective, *lead time is essential*. Nor does it mean that survival analyses and comparison of screen-detected with symptomatic cancers are uninformative: it simply means that they do not prove that screening works in principle.

So how *do* we establish the effectiveness or otherwise of cancer screening interventions in principle? As with most medical interventions, the design of choice is the randomized trial: we randomize one population to receive the intervention (or rather be offered the intervention) and another to usual care. If, as for mammography screening for breast cancer, or fecal occult blood testing for colorectal cancer, the aim is to detect cancer at an early stage and prevent death from the disease, then the appropriate trial endpoint is death from the disease, offset by the total populations randomized to each group, whether the intervention group members took up the offer of screening or not, and regardless of whether the persons randomized developed the cancer in question or not. The time origin should be the point of randomization (not the point of diagnosis of cases, as in survival analysis).

This basic design avoids the classic biases mentioned previously, and as the comparison is of the randomized groups whether or not they were actually screened, it avoids self-selection issues. An example is the Swedish Two-County Trial of mammographic screening. The subjects were randomized to the offer of regular mammography screening, or not, over a period of approximately 7 years, and followed up for a total of 29 years for mortality from breast cancer.[5] Results are shown in **Table 1**. The table shows a significant 31% reduction in breast cancer mortality with the offer of screening. The investigators converted this to an absolute effect of 1 breast cancer death prevented per 1344 mammographic examinations, or per 414 persons screened 3 times over a period of 7 years.[5] We remark that this was the final follow-up of the Two-County Trial, cited here as it is most relevant to the calculation of absolute benefit. The relative benefit has remained constant since the initial publication of mortality results in 1985, which informed screening policy in many coiuntries.[6]

It should be noted that although the randomized trial design as described avoids the anticonservative biases of lead time and length bias, it is inherently conservative. In the first instance, substantial noncompliance with screening dilutes the effect. In the Two-County Trial, compliance was relatively high, approximately 85%, but this still means that the effect of screening is diluted by the 15% who did not receive screening and presumably did not receive any mortality reduction as a result. Thus, although randomized trials measure the efficacy of screening, they often do not provide an

Table 1
Primary result of the Swedish Two-County Trial of mammographic screening at 29-year follow-up

Trial Group	Subjects Randomized	Breast Cancer Deaths	RR (95% Confidence Interval)
Intervention	77,080	351	0.69 (0.56–0.84)
Control	55,985	367	1.00 (−)

Abbreviation: RR, relative risk.

accurate estimate of the effectiveness of screening among the population that actually undergoes screening.

A second issue is that to measure the full benefit of screening, a trial would have to follow up the entire study population to death, which is not feasible and would not deliver a sufficiently timely result. However, there needs to be a minimum follow-up period; put in stark terms, the duration of the trial has to be long enough for cancers in the control group first to come to symptomatic attention and thereafter to cause death. This is illustrated in **Fig. 1**, which shows a cancer in the intervention group of a trial of effective screening, and its equivalent cancer in the control group. In both cases, the tumor is "born" in year 2. In the intervention arm, it is detected before any symptoms by screening in year 4, treated successfully, and the host goes on to live for 21 years afterward and dies of other causes in year 25. In the control group, the corresponding cancer is diagnosed symptomatically in year 7, treatment is unsuccessful and the host dies in year 11. The point is that this represents a cancer death prevented by screening, but with only 10 years of follow-up from randomization it would not be observed. The longer the follow-up, the fewer such unobserved benefits.

There is a related cause of underestimation of benefit. Screening trials in general offer the intervention for a relatively short period of time, usually less than 10 years, and in some cases less than 5.[7] The cancers diagnosed during this screening phase, in both trial groups, are followed up thereafter for death, specifically from the cancer in question. Under the principle of randomization, without any screening, we would expect rates of diagnosis in both trial groups to be parallel over time. However, in the presence of screening in one arm and usual care in the other, some cancers that subsequently cause death are diagnosed in the control group after the end of the screening phase, but during the screening phase in the intervention group due to lead time. Deaths from these cancers will be included in the intervention group but deaths from their counterparts in the control group will not be included. This will bias the result against the screening. Duffy and Smith[8] showed that this bias can be partially corrected by offering an exit screen to the control group contemporaneously with the final screen of the intervention group. This design was used in the Swedish Two-County and Gothenburg Trials.[5,9]

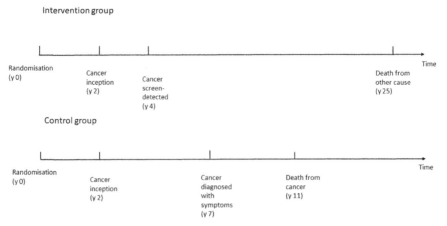

Fig. 1. Illustration of potential timescale of prevention of cancer death in a trial of screening.

When screening for a precursor lesion with the objective of preventing cancer altogether, the randomized trial remains the design of choice. The 2 main differences are that the exit screen of the control group is no longer necessary, and of course the endpoint is cancer diagnosis rather than cancer death, as in the UK Flexible Sigmoidoscopy Trial for prevention of colorectal cancer.[3]

Deaths from Other Causes

It is sometimes argued that screening should show a significant effect on all-cause mortality to inform policy,[10] or it is implied, such as when one reads in a systematic review that a 30% reduction in disease-specific mortality was observed, *"but there was no reduction in all-cause mortality."* Consideration of a simple example shows that the focus on all-cause mortality is ill-considered. Let us take the example of ovarian cancer, which might be responsible for approximately 4% of all deaths in a typical middle-aged female population. Suppose the effect of the offer of ovarian cancer screening is to reduce ovarian cancer mortality by 20%, without affecting deaths from other causes. In a very large trial with 100,000 all-cause deaths expected in the control group, the expected number of deaths in the study group would be 99,200 ($0.04 \times 0.2 \times 100,000 = 800$). Thus, the expected all-cause mortality relative risk would be 0.992 with a 95% confidence interval of 0.9834 to 1.0008; that is, even with 100,000 expected all-cause deaths in each arm, the error bars completely swamp the effect of the screening. A study with 300,000 all-cause deaths expected in each arm would arguably be powered for this effect. Does this mean that to evaluate ovarian cancer screening, we need a trial with 12 million women, 6 million in each arm and follow-up such that 5% in each arm die from any cause? No, it means that the effect of ovarian cancer screening on all-cause mortality is essentially unverifiable. The answer is surely to have cause-specific death from the cancer in question and from the sequelae of screening or treatment for that cancer as the endpoint, and to adopt very rigorous cause of death determination policies, with a high rate of autopsy if necessary.

One can see the absurdity of the advocacy of all-cause mortality if one applies the philosophy in other areas, such as seat belt legislation or road speed restrictions, traveler vaccinations, migrant animal quarantine, and so on.

The use of all-cause mortality is sometimes advocated on the grounds of objectivity. Apart from the fact that human judgment is required in all areas of medicine and health, one might comment that its use discards so many things that we know. These include that only those with a cancer can die of it, only those irradiated can die of a radiation-induced disorder, and so on. The way to effective evaluation is to use our knowledge in trial design, not to throw it away. The evaluator also can use the technique of excess mortality analysis, which compares the excess deaths in cancers diagnosed in the intervention group over the death rate in the population at large, with the corresponding excess morality in cancers diagnosed in the control group, without classifying deaths by cause at all. This was used in the overview of Swedish breast screening trials, and confirmed the reduction in cause-specific mortality.[11]

In noting that all-cause mortality is an inappropriate endpoint in public health interventions generally, Sasieni and Wald[12] acknowledge that the question of whether the intervention under investigation does increase the risk from other causes of death is a valid one. In the first instance we assess whether the screening has the desired effect on the primary endpoint, death or incidence of the cancer in question. It is then reasonable to ask whether the screening is associated with an increased risk of other causes of death. The difficult question is how to elicit this?

First, one would check whether there was a significant or suggestive effect of the intervention on deaths from all other causes than the cancer in question, in the entire population. One might be tempted to do the same for a substantial number of individual causes of death, but this would be mistaken. If one tested 20 causes of death, one would expect one spurious result at the 5% significance level. Instead, consider the preceding remarks about what we know. For example, advocates of use of all-cause mortality for breast screening trials suggest that the reduction in breast cancer deaths may be compensated for by deaths from more frequent use of radiotherapy in screen-detected cancers or as adverse effects of treatment in larger numbers of cancers treated due to larger numbers of cases found in the screened arm.[13] To address this issue, the obvious answer is to compare deaths from other causes between the 2 groups **in the cancer cases only**, or to carry out an excess mortality analysis, as in the Swedish overview.[11]

As a general strategy in a trial of screening to prevent mortality from an individual cancer, we would therefore suggest the following:

1. Compare mortality from the cancer targeted.
2. Compare mortality from all other causes combined.
3. Compare excess mortality from the cancers diagnosed.
4. Testing for differences between groups as a whole in specific causes of death should be done only for plausible, protocol-specified hypotheses.

Other Endpoints Including Overdiagnosis

Other endpoints addressed in screening trials include incidence of the cancer in question, rates of various treatment modalities, and psychological outcomes. It is beyond the scope of this article to specify detailed analyses for these, but some observations should be made here.

One adverse effect of screening that has received considerable attention is overdiagnosis. The most common definition of this is the diagnosis of a histologically confirmed cancer as a result of screening that would not have been diagnosed in the patient's lifetime if screening had not taken place. In the past, this has been estimated by crude comparison of incidence between the intervention and control groups.[13,14] There are major problems with this approach. These include the phenomenon of lead time.[15] An excess may be observed between intervention and control groups, but a portion of this will be due to cases diagnosed in the intervention group whose counterparts in the control group will be diagnosed in the future but have not been diagnosed yet. This portion represents early diagnosis, not overdiagnosis, but it is often included in the latter.

This is eloquently illustrated by the European trial of PSA screening for prostate cancer.[16–18] In this trial, 77,890 men were randomized to periodic PSA testing and 89,353 to usual care. **Table 2** shows incidence results at 11, 13, and 16 years' follow-up. The excess number of cancers in the intervention group reduces over time, as the control group "catches up" by diagnosis of cancers that would have been detected years earlier in the intervention group. It should be noted that the numbers of prostate cancer deaths prevented increases with follow-up time, so that the numbers of excess cases per life saved at the 3 follow-up points are respectively 41, 22, and 18. This illustrates that too short an observation period will underestimate the benefits and overestimate the harms of screening.

This excess due to lead time can also induce an artificial excess in treatment modalities. The implication is not that these comparisons cannot be made, but that they should be either mathematically adjusted for lead time or at the very least, interpreted in the light of lead time.

Table 2 Prostate cancer incidence in the European trials of prostate-specific antigen screening by follow-up time				
Follow-up	Study Group	Subjects	Prostate Cancer Cases (Rate/1000)	Excess Cases in Intervention Group
11 y	Control	89,353	4307 (48)	—
	Intervention	77,890	5990 (77)	2251
13 y	Control	89,353	6107 (68)	—
	Intervention	77,890	7408 (95)	2111
16 y	Control	89,353	7732 (87)	—
	Intervention	77,890	8444 (108)	1668

Also, as noted previously, some trials have an exit screen of the control group. Even when analysis is limited to trials that did not (nominally) screen the control group at the close of the screening phase, and consider long follow-up for which lead time is less of an issue,[14] there remain methodological issues of design of the trials, which detract from the validity of a simple comparison of incidence.[19]

There is a final reason why incidence from the randomized trials may not be useful for estimating absolute rates of overdiagnosis or of cancers treated by certain modalities. The trial populations are unlikely to be representative of the general population targeted for screening by routine services, and due to the timescale issues mentioned previously may be characterized by incidence rates of past decades. Although relative benefits in terms of mortality may usually be generalized, absolute rates of incidence cannot. For further suggestions with respect to overdiagnosis, see the next section.

SERVICE SCREENING EVALUATION

Here we consider the task of assessing whether a routine screening program is delivering the expected benefit, and the estimation of one of the major publicly expressed concerns about screening, overdiagnosis.

Estimation of Benefit

The major benefit of screening is either reduction in mortality from disease, as in breast cancer screening, or reduction in incidence, as in endoscopic screening, aimed at detecting and removing adenomatous polyps to prevent progression to invasive colorectal cancer, or cervical screening, aimed at detecting and removing cervical intraepithelial neoplasia and thus preventing progression to invasive cervical carcinoma. A similar range of observational methodologies is available for both. Essentially there is a choice of cohort or case-control approaches, with different tactical methodological choices available within both.

For cohort approaches, assuming that mortality or incidence can be ascertained, 2 issues have paramount importance. The first is to have a source of a counterfactual estimate of what the mortality or incidence would have been if the screening had not taken place. The second is the need for to ensure accurate ascertainment of exposure to screening.

To obtain counterfactual estimates in a nonrandomized setting, there are sometimes geographic comparator groups available, as when Copenhagen introduced mammography screening before the rest of Denmark.[20] More often, however, data are available only on a single region or country when the screening was introduced universally in a relatively short period. In this case, we have the choice of historical comparison (before-after), or contemporaneous comparison of those accepting the offer of screening with those not doing so. The former is confounded with temporal changes; for example, in treatment of the disease, and the latter is prone to self-selection bias, whereby those who choose to be screened are at different risk of dying of the cancer in question than those who do not. Methods are available to deal with both, including comparison of those unscreened before the screening with those unscreened due to declining the offer of screening in the screening era, and formal mathematical correction for the self-selection bias.[21,22] The main message here is to be aware of these potential biasing features and adopting design or analytical methods to reduce their effect.

For the second issue, the problem is not simply to ensure accurate data on screening invitation and attendance, although this is clearly necessary. It also requires linkage of mortality with data on date of diagnosis. Consider a screening program for prostate cancer that starts in the year 2000 and a prostate cancer death in 2004. The survival figures for prostate cancer mean that in all probability that cancer was diagnosed before 2000, that is, before screening was available. To correctly classify exposure to screening in observational cohorts, a powerful tactic is to define the endpoint as "refined," or incidence-based mortality, that is, deaths from cancers diagnosed *after* the introduction of screening.[22] More recently, an interesting variant on this has been used in both breast and prostate cancer, that is, the incidence of cancers subsequently proving fatal within a certain period of diagnosis.[23,24] This has the added advantage of correctly classifying the exposure status of the population denominator at the relevant time, that is, the diagnosis year, in addition to the exposure status of the cases with the endpoint.

The case-control approach essentially works as follows: cases are persons with the endpoint (for example, death from breast cancer, diagnosis of invasive cervical carcinoma), and controls are persons without the endpoint, matched for age, sex, and opportunity for screening. The cases and matched controls are then compared with respect to screening exposure before the diagnosis dates of the cases. The rationale is that if screening is preventing deaths or diagnoses, the cases will be characterized by lesser screening exposure history than the controls. This design is often less resource-intensive and facilitates straightforward individual classification of screening exposure, but is equally subject to potential self-selection bias and may have other biases related to retrospective identification of cases and ascertainment of exposure.

The case-control evaluation has frequently been used for breast cancer screening,[25] but arguably, the paradigmatic example is the UK case-control evaluation of cervical cancer screening.[26] In this study, 1305 cases of invasive cervical cancer were compared with 2532 age-matched disease-free controls. This study showed no benefit of screening in women younger than 25 and demonstrated a longer-lasting protection of a screen at older ages. This informed the age limits and interscreening intervals in the national program in the United Kingdom. The program changed the lower age limit to 25 and instituted 3-yearly screening for women younger than 50 years old, and 5-yearly for older women.

The case-control approach is therefore an attractive and potentially powerful one. However, researchers adopting this approach should be aware of a number of complicating factors:

- Only screening before the date of diagnosis of the case is relevant. Thus, controls are given a pseudodiagnosis date, equal to the date of diagnosis of their matched case.[26]

- Self-selection bias, and methods for correction for this.[27]
- Screening opportunity bias: if the screen at which a case is detected is included as exposure, the result underestimates the benefit of screening, whereas if it is excluded, the result overestimates the benefit.[28] The true effect will be likely between the two, and a sensitivity analysis may be done by adding a potential lead time to the pseudodiagnosis date of the controls.[29]
- Ascertainment issues: there may be differential identification of cases and controls by screening history. The remedy for this is high-quality cancer registration and screening data, and vigilance against the possibility of ascertainment bias.

Overdiagnosis

Potential adverse effects of screening include discomfort or embarrassment from the test, radiation exposure from the test or subsequent examinations, investigations following suspicious screening results in screenees who turn out not to have cancer, anxiety about cancer, and overdiagnosis. The last of these has received most attention in recent years. As noted previously, a common definition is the diagnosis as a result of screening of cancer that would not have been diagnosed in the host's lifetime if screening had not taken place. Because it is not possible to distinguish histologically a truly nonprogressive cancer from one that is progressive, rates of overdiagnosis commonly are estimated by comparing incidence rates in a group that underwent screening with a group that did not.

With the preceding definition, at least some overdiagnosis must occur in the case of screening to detect frank cancer at an earlier stage. We cannot have successful screening without lead time, and due to competing risks of death from other causes, we cannot have lead time without overdiagnosis. Some who have undergone screening will die shortly thereafter unexpectedly, whereas others' deaths were anticipated, and yet a referral for screening was made without consideration of the lack of potential benefit.

Overdiagnosis can be expressed in several different ways, which will give different impressions to both health professionals and potential screenees.[30] It is probably fair to say, however, that to the cancer scientist, the interesting measure is the proportion of screen-detected cancers that are overdiagnosed, whereas to the person invited to screening and the provider of screening, the more relevant measure is the absolute population risk of an overdiagnosed cancer.

Various approaches have been adopted to estimate overdiagnosis in the context of screening services in routine health care. Many of these depend on comparison of incidence of cancer in the context of a screening program, compared with a counterfactual incidence, estimated from historical data. This has 2 major problems, best considered in the context of mammography screening. The first is that in the late twentieth century, when mammography programs were being set up in many countries, incidence of breast cancer was on the increase because of changes in reproductive behavior, body habitus, and other risk factors. The second is the issue of lead time mentioned previously. Puliti and colleagues[31] showed that studies that failed to take account of these complicating factors obtained high estimates of overdiagnosis and studies that took account of them resulted in low estimates, the latter being more reliable in theory and more plausible in practice.

Another point to note is that when overdiagnosis estimation is driven primarily by incidence of disease, long-term observation is necessary. Consider the example of the prostate screening trial in **Table 2**. The longer the observation period, the smaller the excess. This also can be illustrated by **Fig. 1**. The cancer in the intervention group is clearly not overdiagnosed, because its corresponding cancer in the control group was diagnosed 3 years later. However, if we had only 5 years of observation, the cancer in the intervention group would be considered as excess and potentially overdiagnosed.

It is possible with detailed screening data, to posit a statistical model of overdiagnosis, involving a heterogeneous tumor population regarding capability of progression to symptomatic disease.[32] This, however, is mathematically and computationally complicated, and it is not unusual for the statistical estimation tool to fail to find a plausible or precise estimate.[32]

The important principle to bear in mind is that simple comparison of incidence in a screened (or invited) population with that in an unscreened population, as described previously, is not a valid estimate of overdiagnosis. Accurate estimation requires taking account of underlying incidence trends and lead time, and requires long-term observation.

In the case of screening for precursor lesions, it is not clear that overdiagnosis is a meaningful concept. Many cervical or colorectal precursors would never have become cancer if left untreated, so in that sense it could be argued that they are overdiagnosed. However, the diagnosis of an adenoma in the colon or a case of cervical intraepithelial neoplasia of grade 2 do not incur treatment beyond well-tolerated excision in an outpatient setting, and do not have the same life-changing effects as a diagnosis of cancer. Thus, overdiagnosis in this context is not of significant public health interest.

ASSESSMENT OF QUALITY OF SCREENING
The Screening Test

The primary measures of a screening test's quality are its sensitivity and specificity. These are best shown by example. **Table 3** shows the results of fecal immunochemical testing (FIT) in 3211 subjects with a threshold of 10 μg of hemoglobin per gram of feces.[33] All subjects also underwent colonoscopy, which was treated as the gold standard of diagnosis in this study, and were classified as positive for advanced neoplasia (cancer or advanced adenoma) or not.

The sensitivity of the test is the probability of a positive result in those who actually have the disease. Of the 311 subjects with advanced neoplasia, 163 had a positive FIT result. This gives an estimated sensitivity for FIT at this threshold of 163/311 = 52%.

The specificity of the test is the probability of a negative result in those who truly do not have the disease. Of 2900 subjects free of disease in this study, 2552 had a negative FIT result. Thus the specificity is estimated as 2552/2900 = 88%.

In addition to this, we can calculate the positive predictive value of the test, that is, the proportion of subjects with a screen positive result who actually have the disease. In this case, it is estimated as 163/511 = 32%.

Table 3
Results of fecal immunochemical testing (FIT) in relation to colonoscopy findings

FIT	Colonoscopy Result (Gold Standard)		Total
	No Advanced Neoplasia	Advanced Neoplasia	
< 10 μg/g	2552	148	2700
≥ 10 μg/g	348	163	511
Total	2900	311	3211

Clearly, a good screening test should have both a high sensitivity and a high specificity. The positive predictive value will depend on the prevalence of the disease in the population tested. A higher-risk population will show a higher positive predictive value.

Intuitively, a higher threshold for FIT in the preceding example would improve specificity at a cost of a loss of sensitivity. Similarly, a lower threshold would yield higher sensitivity and lower specificity. When the test can be expressed as a continuum, as in this case, the combined positive and negative accuracy can be described by a receiver operating curve (ROC). This is a plot of the sensitivity against 1-specificity for the points on the continuum. **Fig. 2** shows the ROC curve for estimated risk of lung cancer from the Liverpool Lung Project, which was used to determine eligibility for low-dose computed tomography screening for lung cancer in the UK Lung Screening Trial.[34]

The diagonal line shows what one would expect if the test had no diagnostic value at all. Clearly the closer the curve is to the left-hand side and the top of the area, the closer the sensitivity and specificity are to 100% and the better the test. The accuracy can be summarized by the area below the curve, in this case 0.72, and again, the closer this area is to 1, the better the test. However, the reduction to a single dimension of accuracy is not necessarily useful. If the diagnostic workup is invasive and potentially harmful, or limited by staff capacity, one might require a minimum specificity and tolerate whatever sensitivity this entailed. On the other hand if the consequences of missing a case were crucial, one might specify a minimum sensitivity. In these cases, a single summary statistic of accuracy is not of particular use.

Quality of a Screening Program

A health care provider delivering a screening program will wish to monitor the quality of that program. The parameters monitored may pertain to the diagnostic quality of the

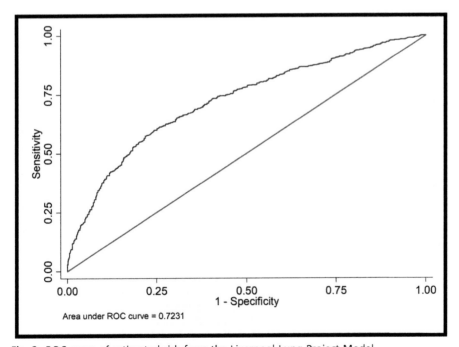

Area under ROC curve = 0.7231

Fig. 2. ROC curve of estimated risk from the Liverpool Lung Project Model.

Table 4
Selected standards and achievable targets for the UK's NHS Breast Screening Program

Parameter	Standard to Be Achieved	Achievable Target
Coverage of target population aged 50–70, %	≥70	≥80
Number referred for assessment (first screen), %	<10	<7
Number referred for assessment (subsequent screens), %	<7	<5
Screen result notification within 2 wk, %	>95	Not stated
Time to assessment within 3 wk, %	>98	100
Benign surgical biopsy rate (first screen)	<1.5/1000	<1/1000
Benign surgical biopsy rate (subsequent screens)	<1/1000	<0.75/1000
Proportion of cancers with preoperative diagnosis, %	≥90	≥95
Standardized cancer detection ratio[a]	>1.00	>1.40
Interval cancers within 12 mo	< 0.65/1000	Not stated

[a] Age-standardized to expected rates from the Swedish Two-County Trial on which the UK program is based.

screening provided, efficiency of the service, or both. **Table 4** shows selected parameters monitored in the UK's National Health Service (NHS) Breast Screening Program, with the standards to be achieved (failure to do so generating remedial action) and achievable targets for units to aim at.[35]

As can be seen, some of the standards are aimed at quality of the screening test (minimum standardized detection ratios), some at quality and acceptability of the program delivered (minimum times to results and assessment appointments), and some to both (maximum percentages recalled for assessment). These are a small sample of many standards applied to the program, which include technical radiographic and radiologic parameters, staging of cancers diagnosed, separate invasive and noninvasive cancer detection rates and standardized detection ratios of invasive cancers of size smaller than 15 mm.

The point of standards such as these is to achieve very high-quality, maximizing benefits and minimizing harms. These are ethically as well as practically important, as screening is not a service requested by the patient. It is offered to the healthy, asymptomatic population as a public health measure, and therefore must be able to guarantee minimum performance for those who take up the offer.

INNOVATIONS TO EXISTING SCREENING PROGRAMS

Diagnostic technology moves faster than the research community can evaluate, thus there is a need for rapid evaluation of innovations in screening practice or technology. As noted previously, the strongest evidence for the efficacy of screening comes from a randomized trial with the clinical endpoint that the screening is intended to prevent as the outcome variable. However, cervical screening has been widespread for decades without such evidence and is generally agreed to have prevented very large numbers of cervical cancer cases and deaths. Also, when proof of principle has been established by one early detection modality, does a potential improvement brought about by a new test need evidence of the same research design?

From changes that have already been made to screening programs, there is an evident consensus that it does not. The changes from film to digital mammography,

Table 5
Detection of 59 cancers by 2D mammography and integrated 2D and DBT in the STORM trial

2D Mammography Result	2D + DBT Result		
	Positive	Negative	Total
Positive	39	0	39
Negative	20	0	20
Total	59	0	59

Abbreviations: DBT, digital breast tomosynthesis; 2D, 2-dimensional.

guaiac fecal testing to immunochemical testing, and from Pap smear to human papillomavirus testing, have all been made in numerous screening programs without the necessity for a randomized trial with death from or incidence of cancer as the endpoint.

When a technological innovation is proposed, there are a number of designs available, but one of the most powerful is the split-sample design, in which all participants receive both the standard screening test and the innovation. The name refers to the use of the design in evaluating a new blood test, in which each participant's blood sample is split into 2 aliquots, 1 to receive the old test, 1 the new. The advantages of this design include the improved precision of within-screenee over between-screenee comparisons, which in turn confers the required statistical power with a smaller study size, and the inbuilt control for personal confounders and center effects. The latter can be particularly important in screening trials in which the participating centers may achieve different screening accuracies.

A good example is the STORM trial of integration of digital breast tomosynthesis (DBT) into breast cancer screening.[36] In this study, 7292 women in Trento and Verona, Italy, were screened with both 2-dimensional digital (2D) mammography, and integrated 2-dimensional mammography and DBT. There were 59 cancers detected. The detection modes of these are shown in **Table 5**. No cancers were detected by 2D mammography alone and not by integrated 2D + DBT. Of the 59 cancers, none were detected by 2D alone, 39 were detected by both modalities, and 20 by integrated 2D + DBT alone.

The formal statistical comparison in this design is between the disagreements, that is, of the 20 cases detected by integrated 2D + DBT alone versus the zero cases detected by 2D alone. This shows a greater detection rate for integrated 2D + DBT, which is highly statistically significant. To achieve 90% statistical power for this difference in detection rates with a comparative trial in which half the subjects received one modality and half the other, would require 37,000 screenees in all, a 5 times greater study size.

Thus, although other designs are available, the split-sample study should always be considered when evaluating new screening technology or other changes to existing programs. It can be incorporated pragmatically within the program, it is fast, efficient, and usually more affordable than alternative designs.

SUMMARY

The preceding has summarized the major considerations and methodological approaches for evaluation of cancer screening. If there is one overriding message for the reader to appreciate, it is that cancer screening evaluation *is not easy*. One cannot approach the subject with only the usual epidemiologic tools. In particular, the shift in the timescale of tumor diagnosis, treatment and potential progression or recurrence adds a degree of complexity to the task. There are, however, clear principles, and sometimes clearly superior approaches, such as the split-sample design for innovations to existing screening programs. However, as in other walks of life, if we find we are getting quick and easy answers, we should always ask ourselves: are we doing something wrong?

REFERENCES

1. Wald NJ. Guidance on terminology. J Med Screen 1994;1:76.
2. Smith RA, Duffy SW, Tabar L. Breast cancer screening: the evolving evidence. Oncology (Willston Park) 2012;26:479–81.
3. Atkin W, Wooldrage K, Parkin DM, et al. Long term effects of once-only flexible sigmoidoscopy screening after 17 years of follow-up: the UK Flexible Sigmoidoscopy Screening randomized controlled trial. Lancet 2017;389(10076):1299–311.
4. Cole P, Morrison AS. Basic issues in population screening for cancer. J Natl Cancer Inst 1980;64:1263–72.
5. Tabar L, Vitak B, Chen THH, et al. Swedish Two-County Trial: impact of mammographic screening on breast cancer mortality during three decades. Radiology 2011;260:658–63.
6. Tabár L, Fagerberg CJ, Gad A, et al. Reduction in mortality from breast cancer after mass screening with mammography. Randomised trial from the Breast Cancer Screening Working Group of the Swedish National Board of Health and Welfare. Lancet 1985;1(8433):829–32.
7. National Lung Screening Trial Research Team, Aberle DR, Adams AM, Berg CD, et al. Reduced lung-cancer mortality with low-dose computed tomographic screening. N Engl J Med 2011;365:395–409.
8. Duffy SW, Smith RA. A note on the design of cancer screening trials. J Med Screen 2015;22:65–8.
9. Bjurstam NG, Björneld LM, Duffy SW. Updated results of the Gothenburg Trial of Mammographic Screening. Cancer 2016;122(12):1832–5.
10. Black WC, Haggstrom DA, Welch HG. All-cause mortality in randomized trials of cancer screening. J Natl Cancer Inst 2002;94(3):167-173.
11. Larsson LG, Nyström L, Wall S, et al. The Swedish randomized mammography screening trials: analysis of their effect on the breast cancer related excess mortality. J Med Screen 1996;3(3):129–32.
12. Sasieni PD, Wald N. Should a reduction in all-cause mortality be the goal when assessing preventive medical therapies? Circulation 2017;135:1985–7.
13. Gøtzsche PC, Jorgensen KJ. Screening for breast cancer with mammography. Cochrane Database Syst Rev 2013;(6):CD001877.
14. Independent UK Panel on Breast Cancer Screening. The benefits and harms of breast cancer screening: an independent review. Lancet 2012;380:1778–86.
15. Duffy SW, Parmar D. Overdiagnosis in breast cancer screening: the importance of length of observation period and lead time. Breast Cancer Res 2013;15:R41.
16. Schröder FH, Hugosson J, Roobol MJ, et al. Prostate-cancer mortality at 11 years of follow-up. N Engl J Med 2012;366:981–90.
17. Schröder FH, Hugosson J, Roobol MJ, et al. Screening and prostate cancer mortality: results of the European Randomized Study of Screening for Prostate Cancer (ERSPC) at 13 years of follow-up. Lancet 2014;384:2027–35.
18. Hugosson J, Roobol MJ, Månsson M, et al. A 16-yr Follow-up of the European Randomized study of Screening for Prostate Cancer. Eur Urol 2019;76(1):43–51.

19. Njor SH, Garne JP, Lynge E. Over-diagnosis estimate from The Independent UK Panel on Breast Cancer Screening is based on unsuitable data. J Med Screen 2013;20:104–5.
20. Olsen AH, Njor SH, Vejborg I, et al. Breast cancer mortality in Copenhagen after introduction of mammography screening: cohort study. BMJ 2005; 330(7485):220.
21. Tabar L, Yen MF, Vitak B, et al. Mammography service screening and mortality in breast cancer patients: 20-year follow-up before and after introduction of screening. Lancet 2003;361:1405–10.
22. Swedish Organised Service Screening Evaluation Group. Reduction in breast cancer mortality from organised service screening with mammography: 1. further confirmation with extended data. Cancer Epidemiol Biomarkers Prev 2006;15(1):45–51.
23. Tabár L, Dean PB, Chen TH, et al. The incidence of fatal breast cancer measures the increased effectiveness of therapy in women participating in mammography screening. Cancer 2019;125:515–23.
24. Kelly SP, Rosenberg PS, Anderson WF, et al. Trends in the incidence of fatal prostate cancer in the United States by race. Eur Urol 2017;71:195–201.
25. Paap E, Verbeek AL, Botterweck AA, et al. Breast cancer screening halves the risk of breast cancer death: a case-referent study. Breast 2014;23:439–44.
26. Sasieni P, Adams J, Cuzick J. Benefit of cervical screening at different ages: evidence from the UK audit of screening histories. Br J Cancer 2003;89:88–93.
27. Duffy SW, Cuzick J, Tabar L, et al. Correcting for non-compliance bias in case-control studies to evaluate cancer screening programs. Appl Stat 2002;51: 235–43.
28. Massat NJ, Dibden A, Parmar D, et al. Impact of screening on breast cancer mortality: the UK program 20 years on. Cancer Epidemiol Biomarkers Prev 2016; 25(3):455–62.
29. Walter SD. Mammographic screening: case-control studies. Ann Oncol 2003; 14(8):1190–2.
30. Njor SH, Paci E, Rebolj M. As you like it: How the same data can support manifold views of overdiagnosis in breast cancer screening. Int J Cancer 2018;143(6): 1287–94.
31. Puliti D, Duffy SW, Miccinesi G, et al, EUROSCREEN Working Group. Overdiagnosis in mammographic screening for breast cancer in Europe: a literature review. J Med Screen 2012;19(Suppl 1):42–56.
32. Ryser MD, Gulati R, Eisenberg MC, et al. Identification of the fraction of indolent tumors and associated overdiagnosis in breast cancer screening trials. Am J Epidemiol 2019;188(1):197–205.
33. Brenner H, Qian J, Werner S. Variation of diagnostic performance of fecal immunochemical testing for hemoglobin by sex and age: results from a large screening cohort. Clin Epidemiol 2018;10:381–9.
34. Field JK, Duffy SW, Baldwin DR, et al. UK Lung Cancer RCT Pilot Screening Trial: baseline findings from the screening arm provide evidence for the potential implementation of lung cancer screening. Thorax 2016;71(2):161–70.
35. Available at: https://assets.publishing.service.gov.uk/government/uploads/system/uploads/attachment_data/file/774770/Breast_draft_standards_V1.7.pdf. Accessed April 9, 2020.
36. Ciatto S, Houssami N, Bernardi D, et al. Integration of 3D digital mammography with tomosynthesis for population breast-cancer screening (STORM): a prospective comparison study. Lancet Oncol 2013;14(7):583–9.

The Development of Cancer Screening Guidelines

Robert A. Smith, PhD

KEYWORDS

- Cancer screening • Guidelines • Evidence-based • Guideline development

KEY POINTS

- Cancer screening guidelines have evolved over the years from being principally expert-driven advice to evidence-driven advice to clinicians, the public, and policy makers.
- Guideline differences are best explained by differences in guideline development methodology, the culture of the guideline developing organization, and the timing of the most recent update.
- Online tools exist to compare guidelines for trustworthiness, and can be used to judge how well a guideline meets Institute of Medicine standards.

INTRODUCTION

In the 1970s, a new generation of clinicians began to challenge conventional medical practice by simply asking, "how do we know this intervention works?" What came to be eventually known as "evidence-based medicine" (EBM)[1] grew from a movement where clinicians were expected to abandon *expert-based medicine*, that is, the practice of medicine based on enduring conventional clinical wisdom and what experts recommended and instead, manage patients based on what the evidence showed was effective. In a published summary of an oral history of EBM organized by the editors of the *Journal of the American Medical Association* and the *British Medical Journal*,[2] Smith and Rennie report this period was defined by the application of increasingly critical appraisal of expert-based medicine, where supporting evidence was sought, and often little was found.[3] During this period, leaders in this movement promoted rigorous research designs, in particular randomized controlled trials (RCTs)[4]; the new field of clinical epidemiology evolved to study clinical practice[4–10]; and organizations dedicated to the systematic evaluation and synthesis of research evidence, such as the Canadian Task Force on Preventive Health Care,[11] the United States Preventive Services Task Force,[12] and The Cochrane Collaboration,[13] were established.

Cancer Screening, Cancer Prevention and Early Detection Department, Center for Cancer Screening, American Cancer Society, 250 Williams Street, Northwest, Suite 600, Atlanta, GA 30303, USA
E-mail address: robert.smith@cancer.org

Med Clin N Am 104 (2020) 955–970
https://doi.org/10.1016/j.mcna.2020.08.009
medical.theclinics.com
0025-7125/20/© 2020 Elsevier Inc. All rights reserved.

In the 1991 editorial where he coined the expression "evidence-based medicine," Guyatt described a scenario where an internist questions the extent of her knowledge in a clinical scenario, conducts a literature search, appraises the citations she receives, and after reviewing the relevant article departs from the clinical course she would have followed had she not sought supporting evidence.[1] The clinician, practicing EBM, used her skills at "literature retrieval, critical appraisal, and information synthesis," which resulted in improved patient care.

As a practical matter, individual clinicians cannot routinely evaluate the literature to ensure the delivery of EBM to the full spectrum of medical care. However, increasingly today's learning pathways are evidence based, and much of basic and on-going modern medical education now is based on applying the principles of EBM to the synthesis of medical information. Clinical practice guidelines (CPGs) serve that same purpose, and with regular updates based on the accumulation of new evidence, existing CPGs can be affirmed or updated. Today, expert groups under the auspices of national health systems and professional societies fulfill that role, ideally following a rigorous methodology to synthesize, assess, and regularly update the clinical and scientific evidence to provide clinicians and the public with recommendations and guidance that is accurate and based on the latest scientific evidence. When patients may wish to make preference-sensitive decisions about undertaking an intervention, decision aids based on these assessments of the evidence of the benefits, limitations, and harms of the intervention can be useful for decision-making.

THE EVOLUTION OF CANCER SCREENING GUIDELINES/RECOMMENDATIONS

The earliest guidance about cancer screening was expert based. Dr. George Papanicolaou devoted many years attempting to persuade clinicians that cytology could be used to diagnose cervical cancer at an early treatable stage. After more than a decade of accumulating evidence, the publication of results in the *American Journal of obstetrics and Gynecology* from a RCT in 1941,[14] and a monograph 2 years later,[15] his ideas, enhanced by the work of others,[16] began to gain widespread acceptance.[17] The American Cancer Society (ACS) had supported Dr. Papanicolaou's research and in 1948 held an interdisciplinary conference to review and promote implementation of cervical cancer screening at a time when pathologists were not persuaded that a malignancy could be identified through the exfoliation of cancer cells.[18–20] In 1957, in what may have been the first cancer screening guideline, the ACS promoted annual screening with the Pap test,[19] and other organizations over time, such as the American College of Obstetricians and Gynecologists, issued similar guidance, with the annual interval very likely chosen for convenience.[17]

According to Winawer, nearly a century ago the concept of the adenoma-carcinoma sequence in the natural history of colorectal cancer was advanced by Lockhart-Mummery and Dukes in 1927,[21] and on-going work at St. Marks Hospital in London in the 1930s demonstrated that patients diagnosed at an earlier stage had better survival. These observations led to efforts to identify colorectal cancer early; although there was speculation that occult bleeding had to be present for some significant duration of time before symptomatic bleeding was apparent, but before the late 1960s, there was no reliable method to detect occult blood. Instead, early efforts to detect colorectal cancer in symptomatic adults focused on rigid sigmoidoscopy. However, in 1948, Gilbertsen and Nelms[22] at the University of Minnesota launched the first screening study based on the concept of detecting occult colorectal cancer in asymptomatic adults using a rigid sigmoidoscope. Although the study methodology had significant limitations, the investigators reported both lower than expected incidence of colorectal cancer and better survival among individuals who had undergone screening. Over time additional studies of sigmoidoscopy were conducted, and in 1961, Day advocated for sigmoidoscopy as part of a cancer detection examination.[23] In 1967 Gregor reported that occult, early stage colorectal cancer could be detected at home using a new guaiac card test (Hemoccult) to detect occult blood[24] and in 1969 endorsed routine testing for the presence of fecal occult blood with the guaiac impregnated cards.[25] By 1974, the ACS was promoting annual stool testing for occult blood in patients older than 40 years, with periodic proctoscopy after age 40 or 50 years (the panel had varying opinions) for adults based on risk and air-contrast barium enema for high-risk patients.[26]

In 1973, encouraging, early results from the Health Insurance Plan (HIP) of Greater New York RCT of breast cancer screening[27] led the ACS and the National Cancer Institute (NCI) to launch the Breast Cancer Detection Demonstration Project (BCDDP). As of 1974, the ACS advised monthly breast self-examination (BSE) beginning at age 21 years, periodic clinical breast examination (CBE), with the interval (6 months–5 years) based on risk (not specified), and periodic mammography for women at high risk.[26] Because early HIP study results for women younger than 50 years were not encouraging, in 1977 a decision was made by the ACS and NCI to restrict BCDDP participation to average-risk women aged 50 years and older and to only offer screening to women younger than 50 years if they were at higher than average risk.[28] This joint statement issued by the ACS and NCI was the first formal breast cancer screening guideline.[29] Annual mammography was recommended for women aged 50 years and older; annual mammography was recommended for women aged 40 to 49 years, only if they had a personal history of breast cancer or a family history of breast cancer (mother or sister); annual screening was recommended for women aged 35 to 39 years if they had a personal history of breast cancer.[29] In addition, the ACS endorsed the importance of periodic CBE and monthly BSE.[29]

In 1980, the ACS adopted a formal evidence-based approach to guideline development that was led by David Eddy, MD, an early leader in the EBM movement, and colleagues at Stanford University.[30] Although prior guidelines had been based on evidence and expert opinion, the lack of methodologic rigor in study designs, the evaluation of the medical literature, and criticism of health screening associated with the growth of EBM led the ACS to subject its current recommendations[26] to the scrutiny of an outside expert who would apply modern principles of EBM to refine the recommendations.[20] The resulting guidelines for the cancer-related checkup were perhaps the very first application of EBM to cancer screening.

A NEW ERA IN GUIDELINE DEVELOPMENT

Since this early period, numerous North American groups have issued cancer screening guidelines for average risk adults, including the ACS, US Preventive Services Task Force (USPSTF), Canadian Task Force on Preventive Health Care, the American College of Physicians (ACP), American Academy of Family Physicians, American College of Radiology, and others. Over time, these groups have tended to adhere to different guideline development methodologies, ranging from little evidence of any systematic methodology to a well-documented, formal process; they have examined different evidence, with different rules for study inclusion and exclusion; and they have brought different values and judgments to assessing the balance of benefits and harms. Different schedules and frequency of updating recommendations also results in guideline differences, mainly due to differences in organizational perspective, methodology, and evidence reviews and guideline updates having taken place in different time periods, with the most recent guideline differing simply because important new evidence had become available. These differences have contributed to a long history of variance in recommendations for cancer screening that has fueled controversies and frustrated policy makers, clinicians, and the target populations.

In 2011, 2 reports from the Institute of Medicine (IOM) established guidelines for systematic evidence reviews and guideline development.[31,32] The reports were motivated by concerns that the proliferation of CPGs had been accompanied by uneven quality, including incomplete inclusion of evidence, inclusion of poor-quality evidence, variable quality in guideline development, lack of transparency, concerns about conflicts of interest among guideline development group members and sponsoring organizations, and the difficulty reconciling conflicting guidelines. At the time of the of IOM publications, there were nearly 2700 CPGs in the Agency for Health Care Research's (AHRQ) National Guidelines Clearinghouse.[32] These 2 reports represented not only guidance for guideline development but also new benchmarks for evaluating the trustworthiness, transparency, and rigor of an evidence-based guideline. In 2011, the ACS also revised its guideline development process to be adherent with the IOM recommendations.[33]

The IOM outlined 8 principles and procedures for developing trustworthy CPGs, which are show in **Table 1** and outlined below in greater detail.[32]

Transparency

The importance of transparency is to ensure that the guideline development process, including the systematic review methodology, protocols, rules for decision-making,

Table 1 Institute of Medicine standards for developing trustworthy clinical practice guidelines	
Standards	**IOM Recommendations**
Transparency	The process and funding of guideline development should be completely specified.
Conflicts of interest	Conflicts of interest include commercial, institutional, professional, and intellectual conflicts, all of which must be openly declared. Members should divest conflicting financial relationships.
Group composition	The guideline group should include multidisciplinary methodological experts, clinicians, and patient advocates.
Systematic review of evidence	The guidelines should be based on a systematic literature review that meets the standards set by the IOM.
Grading strength of recommendations	For each recommendation, the text should explain the evidence and the reasoning, the balance of benefits and harms, and should indicate the level of confidence in the recommendation.
Articulation of recommendations	Recommendations should be clearly stated and actionable.
External review	The draft guidelines should be posted for public comment, and the final guidelines should be revised as appropriate before peer review.
Updating	Guidelines should be updated when new evidence could result in modifying the recommendations.

Data from Institute of Medicine. Clinical Practice Guidelines We Can Trust. . Washington, DC: National Academies Press; 2011.

disclosures and real or potential conflicts of interest, sources of funding support, etc. are clearly and completely disclosed; in other words, who developed the guideline and the process by which it was derived. The IOM also stressed that it was important to explain the rules for inclusion and exclusion of evidence, how the data were interpreted, the basis for assessing the magnitude of the benefits and harms, and the basis for judgments about the balance of benefits and harms.[32]

Conflicts of Interest and Group Composition

In 2009, the IOM defined a conflict of interest (COI) as "A set of circumstances that creates a risk that professional judgment or actions regarding a primary interest will be unduly influenced by a secondary interest."[34] Note that the IOM did not state that the circumstances *would* create a COI, only that they *could* create a COI. In this respect, the common label of any interest as a COI creates a defensive situation where the participant must regard an interest and a COI as equivalent, as both an actual COI or the perception of a COI are treated as the same for purposes of avoiding suspicion that the guideline was not trustworthy.

Potential COIs may be financial, professional (the latter may be intertwined), institutional, or ideological. Financial COI occur when income is directly tied to guideline issues, that is, clinical services, industry-sponsored research, investments, consulting, etc. These COI may exist with individuals or the organization sponsoring the development of the guideline. With professional COIs, decisions about utilization of a screening tests may be perceived as going beyond evidence to promote greater use of a screening technology, which may also be perceived as a financial COI. This judgment does not presume that COI is inherent, only that it may be, and even if there is only the perception of a COI, confidence in the trustworthiness of a guideline can be diminished. Institutional COI may occur when a guideline panel member is associated with an organization with an interest in the guideline topic, or an institutional COI may exist if the organization developing the guideline has a financial relationship with commercial entities with an interest in the guideline outcome. A shortcoming of the IOM statement on COI in guideline development is the neglect of professional specialization or ideological bias where there is no direct or indirect potential for financial gain. A professional specialization may also be associated with a bias for or against screening, or an individual may have an ideological bias associated with a career-long orientation that has been unwavering in support or lack of support for screening.

Management of COI was a cornerstone of the IOM report on the development of trustworthy guidelines,[32] although the recommendations do not entirely overcome the tradeoffs between avoiding real or potential COI and the need for the clinical expertise of specialists. The IOM report cited strategies taken by some organizations to address COI, including omission from guideline development panels for any COI, a financial threshold, balancing membership in a guideline panel to minimize the number of members with COI, and allowing participation, but requiring recusal from specific deliberations and/or decision-making. The IOM report recommended that before selection of a guideline development panel, potential members should disclose "all current and planned commercial (including services from which a clinician derives a substantial proportion of income), noncommercial, intellectual, institutional, and patient–public activities pertinent to the potential scope of the CPG."[32] The IOM report concluded that when possible, guideline development panel members should not have any COIs. However, the IOM recognized that exclusion of experts because of COI could leave a panel without needed expertise and recommended that experts with COI should be a minority of members and that chairs and co-chairs of the panel should not have any COIs.[32] Although this recommendation seems straightforward enough, it is not entirely feasible for a specialty organization that wishes to develop a clinical practice guideline and avoid *all* potential COI. It is not realistic to expect that a specialty organization would recruit a nonspecialist panel from outside the organization to develop their guideline, so a reasonable approach to avoiding COI can be based on recruiting some nonconflicted methodologists to be on the guideline development panel, with remaining members being specialists with minimum COI (ie, excluding members with investments, significant consulting relationships, etc.).

As a real-world example, the ACS approach to COI includes full disclosure of all potential financial, professional, institutional, and ideological COI, for which the latter includes a history of academic writing and presentations that are pertinent to a guideline under development. These disclosure statements are reviewed to determine if any interests are determined to represent a concerning level of real or potential or perceived COI. If so, the guideline development group member will be asked to recuse themselves from the development of the guideline. All disclosures are included as an appendix to the final guideline article. The ACS also separates the process of receiving expert input from the process determining the guideline and writing the guideline. Members of the ACS guideline development group include one patient advocate, and the remaining 11 members are generalist health care professionals and primary care physicians with expertise in the interpretation of evidence regarding benefits, limitations, and harms of clinical interventions, with some members having experience in the evaluation of screening. For each new guideline, the ACS establishes an expert advisory committee who are asked to consult with the guideline development panel on a regular basis and review draft protocols and systematic review methodology and early and final drafts of the guideline. This approach provides the guideline writing group with appropriate specialty expertise while also protecting it from the appearance of specialty COI.

Systematic Evidence Review

A systematic review of relevant evidence is an essential component of a credible, trustworthy guideline development process, and the companion report to *Clinical Practice Guidelines We Can Trust*[32] was *Finding What Works in Health Care: Standards for Systematic Reviews*.[31] The IOM defines a systematic review as "a scientific investigation that focuses on a specific question and uses explicit, preplanned scientific methods to identify, select, assess, and summarize the findings of individual, relevant studies."[31] The same principles described earlier for ensuring transparency and trustworthiness by avoiding bias and COI also apply to systematic evidence reviews. First, it is important to avoid bias and COI in the choice of the review team, and second, the systematic review must be guided by a detailed methodology for identification of evidence, criteria for inclusion and exclusion of evidence, and how the evidence will be evaluated. The IOM report summarizes (1) standards for initiating a systematic review, which mostly pertain to defining the scope of the topic and developing the protocol; (2) standards for literature searches and critical appraisal of studies; (3) standards for synthesizing the body of evidence; (4) standards for reporting the results of systematic reviews; and (5) issues related to the relationship between the systematic review team and the guideline writing panel. With respect to the relationship between the review team and the writing panel, the IOM describes various degrees of interaction, ranging from complete isolation of the systematic review team from the guideline development panel to the guideline development panel conducting the systematic review and writing the guideline. Although the IOM report tends to favor more versus less isolation between the 2 groups, there is clear value to some interaction to ensure that the final systematic review meets the needs of the guideline development panel.

Perhaps the best-known example of this process are the systematic evidence reviews conducted for the USPSTF by the AHRQ Evidence-Based Practice Centers. These systematic reviews are the basis for the USPSTF's assessment of the scientific evidence for clinical preventive services. A condensed version of the review usually accompanies the publication of the recommendation statement. Systematic reviews are archived in the National Library of Medicine and can be accessed at https://www.ncbi.nlm.nih.gov/books/NBK43437/. These reviews generally accompany the recommendations. The USPSTF updated their methods for evidence reviews and recommendation development in 2007.[35]

Grading the Strength of the Evidence and Recommendations

It has become increasingly accepted that a key methodological element of a high-quality clinical practice guideline is an assessment of the quality of the evidence, which is tied to the strength of the recommendation. Ultimately, the strength of the recommendation reflects the possibility that new evidence might result in a different recommendation, the degree of certainty that desirable outcomes outweigh undesirable outcomes, and the degree of confidence that all patients would accept the intervention as worth undertaking.

The assessment of the quality of the evidence essentially is a measure of the confidence in the conclusions derived from the appraisal of the evidence. This degree of confidence is linked to research designs, which means that the highest quality evidence derives from RCTs, followed by controlled trials without randomization, cohort studies or case-control studies, and uncontrolled case series. Each of these methodologies must also be assessed for the quality of their design, sample size, etc., to arrive at an overall quality rating. In a well-designed systematic review, if a study is accepted for initial inclusion, at least 2 individuals independently will rate the quality of the study, and if there is disagreement, a final determination will be reached by consensus or by another reviewer. Studies will then receive a score (1–4, with subdivisions), a rating (good, fair, poor), or a letter grade (A, B, C). Other factors that may be considered in the overall assessment of the evidence are the generalizability of the studies, number of good-quality studies, and consistency of the findings in the literature. Rating evidence is intended to ensure that studies receive systematic scrutiny, study strengths and weaknesses are identified, and subjectivity is minimized. Still, as would be expected, there is considerable subjectivity and variation in judgment about the strength of evidence, even when using the same system, and quite often a key step in a systematic evidence review that is intended to convey transparency, that is, how judgments about study quality were reached, is not transparent at all.

The most common system for grading evidence and recommendations is the Grades of Recommendation, Assessment, Development, and Evaluation (GRADE), which is used by more than 100 organizations in 19 countries.[36,37] GRADE shares a common feature with most grading systems in that the system of evidence grading, and the strength of the recommendation highly depends on the ranking of the study methodology. Most of these systems were designed to evaluate therapeutic interventions in individuals who are being treated for a condition, and thus ideally there should be a sufficient number of RCTs from which to assess the efficacy of the intervention. In contrast, there are very few RCTs of screening, they vary considerably in their quality, and may reflect older technology and protocols. Because new RCTs are unlikely to be funded, and would face ethical challenges anyway, modern evaluations of screening will be carried out with observational studies. Further, initial trials will be conducted in average risk populations, with demonstrations of efficacy applied to higher risk populations, for which RCTs are especially difficult. This means that under these grading systems, most of the study designs are inherently judged to be of moderate to low quality (typically "low"), and the strength of the recommendations rarely qualify as "strong;" rather, the next recommendation rating in the scale is "weak," although it is acceptable to substitute "qualified." A weak recommendation means "trade-offs [between benefits and harms] are less certain, either because of low-quality evidence or because evidence suggests that desirable and undesirable effects are closely balanced."[32] Essentially, when using the GRADE system, even against the backdrop of evidence from RCTs, a very well-designed observational study that has favorable findings usually will be judged as low- or moderate-quality evidence, resulting in a weak recommendation. GRADE does allow for a strong recommendation if the study is well designed and there is a clear dose-response relationship or a large observed effect, but it seems clear that in practice, a strong evidence grade is limited for RCTs. Observational studies commonly are judged to be second-class citizens. Although guideline developers understand that their recommendation carries the full confidence of the issuing organization that the intervention is recommended fully and not with hesitation, referring physicians and patients may interpret the recommendation language as conveying low confidence. This is a situation that must be the focus of further attention in guideline development methodology.

Articulation of Benefits and Harms

Guideline developers are expected to assess the evidence for harms associated with screening, and there is an expectation that there should be an assessment of whether benefits outweigh harms. This assessment may be associated with considerable subjectivity. Challenges include the comparison of different data sources, that is, intention-to-treat effects of benefit from a meta-analysis versus observational data from adults all of whom were exposed to the intervention. It is also clear that benefits associated with screening, such as avoiding a diagnosis of an advanced breast cancer or death from breast cancer, are very different metrics compared with being recalled for further imaging or undergoing a biopsy. Studies of harms may also have subjective elements in their methodology not easily discerned by the systematic review team, who may place greater scrutiny on study methodology influences on estimates of benefit than they do on studies of harms. It should be understood that subjectivity is unavoidable in the assessment of the balance of benefits and harms, and thus what is important is clear articulation of the basis for subjective judgments. For example, the USPSTF places strong emphasis on the recall rate and estimates of overdiagnosis as important harms in breast cancer screening.[38] In contrast, the ACS stated that it did not regard being recalled for further evaluation as an important harm, and although overdiagnosis was judged to be an important harm, the data were insufficient to estimate the magnitude of overdiagnosis as a harm with any measurable confidence.[39]

External Review

Once a guideline is developed, there is value in subjecting it to external review from subject-matter experts (including those who may have been advisors during the guideline development process), likely guideline advocates as well as likely detractors, and key stakeholder organizations that represent a broad spectrum of positions. The ACS and the USPSTF each subjects their draft guidelines to external review before finalization, and these reviews not only have resulted in changes in narrative to improve clarity but in a few instances external reviews have resulted in significant changes in the recommendation statements.

In addition to feedback on the guideline or recommendation, external reviewers may identify small details that require correction, logic that is unclear and poorly explained, or gaps in logic and flaws in methodology. Reviewers may identify flaws in the underlying evidence for a recommendation that may appropriately weaken the strength of the recommendation. External reviewers may identify implications and consequences of a new guideline or guideline change that may not have been anticipated or fully appreciated. The review period should be regarded as a key opportunity to correct errors, improve the narrative, and even rethink a recommendation. It provides an opportunity for the guideline development panel to reflect on the entirety of their effort and to be sure that the guideline development process and the recommendations stand up to scrutiny. To be sure, some feedback may be inflammatory, baseless and ideological, and thus entirely useless other than providing a preview to how an organization will respond publicly to the new guideline once it is released. However, it is important to remember that guideline development is a rather insular endeavor; guideline implementation takes a village, and thus feedback from end-users is a valuable step in the process.

Guideline Updates

At the most basic level, a clinical practice guideline should reflect the current state of the evidence. Clinicians, policy makers, and the public expect that a guideline reflects the most up-to-date evidence and reasonably expect that when it does not, it will be updated. Shekelle and colleagues[40] outlined 6 situations that should lead to updating a guideline: a change in evidence related to benefits and harms; a change in important outcomes; a change in available interventions; a change in evidence that current practice is optimal; a change in values placed on outcomes (benefits or harms); and a change in available resources.

Given that guideline development is a major investment in time and resources, and more now than ever given the IOM guidance, a guideline should be updated periodically, and in the interim, there should be periodic reassurance that the current guideline still reflects best practice. If not, there should be public notice that an update is underway. The IOM emphasized the following best practices to reflect the currency of an existing guideline and considerations for periodic updates. First, a guideline must clearly identify the period from which the existing evidence is drawn. Second, the scientific literature must be monitored to identify relevant new evidence that could alter existing recommendations or reaffirm the current recommendation. Third, when new evidence may lead to a modification of the current guideline (new technology, new evidence related to the intervention protocol, new evidence on harms, or modification of the target population), a guideline update process should be initiated.[32]

GUIDELINE EVALUATION

Despite an extensive and growing literature on systematic reviews and guideline development, CPGs still vary in quality, and it is difficult for users of guidelines to scrutinize the lengthy checklist of esoteric criteria that determines where a guideline lands on a scale of trustworthiness. The ECRI Guidelines Trust evaluates registered guidelines for trustworthiness, applying a TRUST (**T**ransparency and **R**igor **U**sing **S**tandards of **T**rustworthiness) scorecard based on IOM standards.[41,42] These scores are available for most guidelines on their Website.[42] An additional tool for addressing the

Table 2
AGREE reporting checklist, 2016

AGREE Reporting Checklist
2016

AGREE
REPORTING CHECKLIST

This checklist is intended to guide the reporting of clinical practice guidelines.

CHECKLIST ITEM AND DESCRIPTION	REPORTING CRITERIA	Page #
DOMAIN 1: SCOPE AND PURPOSE		
1. OBJECTIVES *Report the overall objective(s) of the guideline. The expected health benefits from the guideline are to be specific to the clinical problem or health topic.*	☐ Health intent(s) (i.e., prevention, screening, diagnosis, treatment, etc.) ☐ Expected benefit(s) or outcome(s) ☐ Target(s) (e.g., patient population, society)	
2. QUESTIONS *Report the health question(s) covered by the guideline, particularly for the key recommendations.*	☐ Target population ☐ Intervention(s) or exposure(s) ☐ Comparisons (if appropriate) ☐ Outcome(s) ☐ Health care setting or context	
3. POPULATION *Describe the population (i.e., patients, public, etc.) to whom the guideline is meant to apply.*	☐ Target population, sex and age ☐ Clinical condition (if relevant) ☐ Severity/stage of disease (if relevant) ☐ Comorbidities (if relevant) ☐ Excluded populations (if relevant)	
DOMAIN 2: STAKEHOLDER INVOLVEMENT		
4. GROUP MEMBERSHIP *Report all individuals who were involved in the development process. This may include members of the steering group, the research team involved in selecting and reviewing/rating the evidence and individuals involved in formulating the final recommendations.*	☐ Name of participant ☐ Discipline/content expertise (e.g., neurosurgeon, methodologist) ☐ Institution (e.g., St. Peter's hospital) ☐ Geographical location (e.g., Seattle, WA) ☐ A description of the member's role in the guideline development group	
5. TARGET POPULATION PREFERENCES AND VIEWS *Report how the views and preferences of the target population were sought/considered and what the resulting outcomes were.*	☐ Statement of type of strategy used to capture patients'/publics' views and preferences (e.g., participation in the guideline development group, literature review of values and preferences) ☐ Methods by which preferences and views were sought (e.g., evidence from literature, surveys, focus groups) ☐ Outcomes/information gathered on patient/public information ☐ How the information gathered was used to inform the guideline development process and/or formation of the recommendations	
6. TARGET USERS *Report the target (or intended) users of the guideline.*	☐ The intended guideline audience (e.g. specialists, family physicians, patients, clinical or institutional leaders/administrators) ☐ How the guideline may be used by its target audience (e.g., to inform clinical decisions, to inform policy, to inform standards of care)	

(continued on next page)

Table 2
(*continued*)

DOMAIN 3: RIGOUR OF DEVELOPMENT		
7. SEARCH METHODS *Report details of the strategy used to search for evidence.*	☐ Named electronic database(s) or evidence source(s) where the search was performed (e.g., MEDLINE, EMBASE, PsychINFO, CINAHL) ☐ Time periods searched (e.g., January 1, 2004 to March 31, 2008) ☐ Search terms used (e.g., text words, indexing terms, subheadings) ☐ Full search strategy included (e.g., possibly located in appendix)	
8. EVIDENCE SELECTION CRITERIA *Report the criteria used to select (i.e., include and exclude) the evidence. Provide rationale, where appropriate.*	☐ Target population (patient, public, etc.) characteristics ☐ Study design ☐ Comparisons (if relevant) ☐ Outcomes ☐ Language (if relevant) ☐ Context (if relevant)	
9. STRENGTHS & LIMITATIONS OF THE EVIDENCE *Describe the strengths and limitations of the evidence. Consider from the perspective of the individual studies and the body of evidence aggregated across all the studies. Tools exist that can facilitate the reporting of this concept.*	☐ Study design(s) included in body of evidence ☐ Study methodology limitations (sampling, blinding, allocation concealment, analytical methods) ☐ Appropriateness/relevance of primary and secondary outcomes considered ☐ Consistency of results across studies ☐ Direction of results across studies ☐ Magnitude of benefit versus magnitude of harm ☐ Applicability to practice context	
10. FORMULATION OF RECOMMENDATIONS *Describe the methods used to formulate the recommendations and how final decisions were reached. Specify any areas of disagreement and the methods used to resolve them.*	☐ Recommendation development process (e.g., steps used in modified Delphi technique, voting procedures that were considered) ☐ Outcomes of the recommendation development process (e.g., extent to which consensus was reached using modified Delphi technique, outcome of voting procedures) ☐ How the process influenced the recommendations (e.g., results of Delphi technique influence final recommendation, alignment with recommendations and the final vote)	
11. CONSIDERATION OF BENEFITS AND HARMS *Report the health benefits, side effects, and risks that were considered when formulating the recommendations.*	☐ Supporting data and report of benefits ☐ Supporting data and report of harms/side effects/risks ☐ Reporting of the balance/trade-off between benefits and harms/side effects/risks ☐ Recommendations reflect considerations of both benefits and harms/side effects/risks	
12. LINK BETWEEN RECOMMENDATIONS AND EVIDENCE *Describe the explicit link between the recommendations and the evidence on which they are based.*	☐ How the guideline development group linked and used the evidence to inform recommendations ☐ Link between each recommendation and key evidence (text description and/or reference list) ☐ Link between recommendations and evidence summaries and/or evidence tables in the results section of the guideline	

(*continued on next page*)

Table 2
(continued)

13. EXTERNAL REVIEW *Report the methodology used to conduct the external review.*	☐ Purpose and intent of the external review (e.g., to improve quality, gather feedback on draft recommendations, assess applicability and feasibility, disseminate evidence) ☐ Methods taken to undertake the external review (e.g., rating scale, open-ended questions) ☐ Description of the external reviewers (e.g., number, type of reviewers, affiliations) ☐ Outcomes/information gathered from the external review (e.g., summary of key findings) ☐ How the information gathered was used to inform the guideline development process and/or formation of the recommendations (e.g., guideline panel considered results of review in forming final recommendations)
14. UPDATING PROCEDURE *Describe the procedure for updating the guideline.*	☐ A statement that the guideline will be updated ☐ Explicit time interval or explicit criteria to guide decisions about when an update will occur ☐ Methodology for the updating procedure
DOMAIN 4: CLARITY OF PRESENTATION	
15. SPECIFIC AND UNAMBIGUOUS RECOMMENDATIONS *Describe which options are appropriate in which situations and in which population groups, as informed by the body of evidence.*	☐ A statement of the recommended action ☐ Intent or purpose of the recommended action (e.g., to improve quality of life, to decrease side effects) ☐ Relevant population (e.g., patients, public) ☐ Caveats or qualifying statements, if relevant (e.g., patients or conditions for whom the recommendations would not apply) ☐ If there is uncertainty about the best care option(s), the uncertainty should be stated in the guideline
16. MANAGEMENT OPTIONS *Describe the different options for managing the condition or health issue.*	☐ Description of management options ☐ Population or clinical situation most appropriate to each option
17. IDENTIFIABLE KEY RECOMMENDATIONS *Present the key recommendations so that they are easy to identify.*	☐ Recommendations in a summarized box, typed in bold, underlined, or presented as flow charts or algorithms ☐ Specific recommendations grouped together in one section
DOMAIN 5: APPLICABILITY	
18. FACILITATORS AND BARRIERS TO APPLICATION *Describe the facilitators and barriers to the guideline's application.*	☐ Types of facilitators and barriers that were considered ☐ Methods by which information regarding the facilitators and barriers to implementing recommendations were sought (e.g., feedback from key stakeholders, pilot testing of guidelines before widespread implementation) ☐ Information/description of the types of facilitators and barriers that emerged from the inquiry (e.g., practitioners have the skills to deliver the recommended care, sufficient equipment is not available to ensure all eligible members of the

(continued on next page)

Table 2
(continued)

	population receive mammography) ☐ How the information influenced the guideline development process and/or formation of the recommendations
19. IMPLEMENTATION ADVICE/TOOLS *Provide advice and/or tools on how the recommendations can be applied in practice.*	☐ Additional materials to support the implementation of the guideline in practice. For example: ☐ Guideline summary documents ☐ Links to check lists, algorithms ☐ Links to how-to manuals ☐ Solutions linked to barrier analysis (see Item 18) ☐ Tools to capitalize on guideline facilitators (see Item 18) ☐ Outcome of pilot test and lessons learned
20. RESOURCE IMPLICATIONS *Describe any potential resource implications of applying the recommendations.*	☐ Types of cost information that were considered (e.g., economic evaluations, drug acquisition costs) ☐ Methods by which the cost information was sought (e.g., a health economist was part of the guideline development panel, use of health technology assessments for specific drugs, etc.) ☐ Information/description of the cost information that emerged from the inquiry (e.g., specific drug acquisition costs per treatment course) ☐ How the information gathered was used to inform the guideline development process and/or formation of the recommendations
21. MONITORING/ AUDITING CRITERIA *Provide monitoring and/or auditing criteria to measure the application of guideline recommendations.*	☐ Criteria to assess guideline implementation or adherence to recommendations ☐ Criteria for assessing impact of implementing the recommendations ☐ Advice on the frequency and interval of measurement ☐ Operational definitions of how the criteria should be measured
DOMAIN 6: EDITORIAL INDEPENDENCE	
22. FUNDING BODY *Report the funding body's influence on the content of the guideline.*	☐ The name of the funding body or source of funding (or explicit statement of no funding) ☐ A statement that the funding body did not influence the content of the guideline
23. COMPETING INTERESTS *Provide an explicit statement that all group members have declared whether they have any competing interests.*	☐ Types of competing interests considered ☐ Methods by which potential competing interests were sought ☐ A description of the competing interests ☐ How the competing interests influenced the guideline process and development of recommendations

From Brouwers MC, Kerkvliet K, Spithoff K, on behalf of the AGREE Next Steps Consortium. The AGREE Reporting Checklist: a tool to improve reporting of clinical practice guidelines. BMJ 2016;352:i1152. Available at: https://www.ncbi.nlm.nih.gov/pmc/articles/PMC5118873/. With permission.

variability in guideline quality and measuring the thoroughness and trustworthiness of a CPG is the Appraisal of Guidelines for Research and Evaluation (AGREE II) instrument, which measures 23 items in 6 quality domains, including (1) scope and purpose, (2) stakeholder involvement, (3) rigor of development, (4) clarity of presentation, (5) applicability, and (6) editorial independence (**Table 2**).[43] The ACP issues CPG updates by reviewing CPGs from other organizations and scrutinizing them with the AGREE II instrument.[44,45]

SUMMARY

The IOM reports that standards for systematic reviews and guideline development were prompted by a growing body of evidence revealing serious shortcomings in transparency and trustworthiness in the development of CPGs. Some organizations may have met these standards, but they were poorly documented; others had serious deficiencies ranging from glaring neglect of COI to weak scientific justification of recommendations. The IOM standards and the Appraisal of Guidelines Research and Evaluation (AGREE)[43] checklist each provides sound guidance for ensuring that a clinical practice guideline is credible, trustworthy, and can measure up to scrutiny. However, these recommendations should be regarded as a yardstick for both best practices and how the guideline may be assessed by outside groups. Ransohoff and colleagues[46] published a commentary on the new standards for trustworthiness that acknowledged the importance of the new standard, but rightfully pointed out that they mostly represented consensus judgments rather than practices based on evidence of their value, and that although well intentioned, they truly imposed an impractical and inflexible standard for trustworthiness. Ransohoff and colleagues[46] cited a recent study[47] that showed poor adherence to the new IOM standards among 114 clinical practice guidelines. Having failed to meet the new standards, were they all untrustworthy?

Guideline development methodology will continue to evolve. It is important to recognize that guidelines differ not only due to variations in guideline development methodology, including not only what evidence is included in the guideline review, but how it is interpreted, but also the judgment that a guideline developing group brings to interpretations about the balance of benefits and harms. What is essential in producing a trustworthy guideline is that both the process and the values and judgments that are the basis for the recommendations are clearly described.

DISCLOSURES

The work was supported by the American Cancer Society.

REFERENCES

1. Guyatt G. Evidence-based medicine. ACP J Club 1991;A-16.
2. Evidence-based medicine: an oral history. JAMA Network. 2018. Available at: https://ebm.jamanetwork.com/. Accessed July 19, 2020.
3. Smith R, Rennie D. Evidence-based medicine–an oral history. JAMA 2014;311: 365–7.
4. Wilson JMG, Jungner G. Principles and practice of screening for disease. Geneva (Switzerland): World Health Organization; 1968.
5. Feinstein AR. Boolean algebra and clinical taxonomy. I. analytic synthesis of the general spectrum of a human disease. N Engl J Med 1963;269:929–38.
6. Feinstein AR. Scientific methodology in clinical medicine. i. introduction, principles, and concepts. Ann Intern Med 1964;61:564–79.
7. Cochrane AL. Effectiveness and efficiency: random reflections on health services. London (United Kingdom).: Nuffield Provincial Hospitals Trust; 1972.
8. Sackett DL. How to read clinical journals, I: why to read them and how to start reading them critically. Can Med Assoc J 1981;124:555–8.
9. Feinstein AR. Clinical epidemiology : the architecture of clinical research. Amsterdam (the Netherlands): Elsevier - Health Sciences Division; 1985.

10. Sackett DL, Haynes RB, Guyatt GH, et al. Clinical epidemiology: a basic science for clinical medicine. 2nd edition. Boston: Little Brown; 1991.

11. History of the Canadian task force on preventive health care. 2019. Available at: https://canadiantaskforce.ca/about/history/. Accessed July 19, 2020.

12. About the USPSTF. Agency for Healthcare Research and Quality. 2020. Available at: https://www.uspreventiveservicestaskforce.org/uspstf/about-uspstf. Accessed July 19, 2020.

13. Cochrane. 2020. Available at: https://www.cochrane.org. Accessed July 19, 2020.

14. Papanicolaou GN. The diagostic value of vaginal sears in carcinoma of the uterus. A J Obstet Gynecol 1941;42:193–206.

15. Papanicolaou GN, Traut HF. Diagnosis of uterine cancer by the vaginal smear. New York: Commonwealth Fund; 1943.

16. Ayre JE, Chevalier PM, Ayre WB. A comparative study of vaginal and cervical cornification in human subjects. J Clin Endocrinol Metab 1947;7:749–52.

17. Waxman AG. Guidelines for cervical cancer screening: history and scientific rationale. Clin Obstet Gynecol 2005;48:77–97.

18. Breslow L. A history of cancer control in the US with emphasis on the period 1946-1971. Los Angeles (CA): University of California at Los Angeles School of Public Health; 1977.

19. Eddy D. Cervical Cancer Screening. CA Cancer J Clin 1980;30:215–23.

20. Gusberg SB. The Role of Guidelines for Cancer Screening. In: Mettlin C, Murphy GP, editors. Progress in clinical and biological research: issues in cancer screening and communication. New York: Alan R. Liss, Inc.; 1982. p. 25–32.

21. Lockhart-Mummery JP, Dukes C. The precancerous changes in the rectum and colon. Surg Gynecol Obstet 1927;36:591–6.

22. Gilbertsen VA, Nelms JM. The prevention of invasive cancer of the rectum. Cancer 1978;41:1137–9.

23. Day E. The cancer detection examination. CA Cancer J Clin 1961;11:103–6.

24. Greegor DH. Diagnosis of large-bowel cancer in the asymptomatic patient. JAMA 1967;201:943–5.

25. Greegor DH. Detection of silent colon cancer in routine examination. CA Cancer J Clin 1969;19:330–7.

26. American Cancer Society. Summary of recommendations for early detection. Cancer 1974;33:1759–61.

27. Strax P, Venet L, Shapiro S. Value of mammography in reduction of mortality from breast cancer in mass screening. Am J roentgenol radium Ther Nucl Med 1973; 117:686–9.

28. National Cancer Institute. National Institutes of Health/National Cancer Institute consensus development meeting on breast cancer screening: issues and recommendations. J Natl Cancer Inst 1978;60:1519–21.

29. Dodd GD. American cancer society guidelines on screening for breast cancer. An overview. Cancer 1992;69:1885–7.

30. Eddy D. ACS report on the cancer-related health checkup. CA Cancer J Clin 1980;30:193–240.

31. Institute of Medicine. Finding what works in health care: standards for systematic reviews. Washington, DC: National Academies Press; 2011.

32. Institute of Medicine. Clinical practice guidelines we can Trust. Washington, DC: National Academies Press; 2011.

33. Brawley O, Byers T, Chen A, et al. New American cancer society process for creating trustworthy cancer screening guidelines. JAMA 2011;306:2495–9.

34. Institute of Medicine. Conflicts of interest in medical research, education, and practice. Washington, DC.: National Academies Press; 2009.
35. Guirguis-Blake J, Calonge N, Miller T, et al. Current processes of the U.S. preventive services task force: refining evidence-based recommendation development. Ann Intern Med 2007;147:117–22.
36. Atkins D, Eccles M, Flottorp S, et al. Systems for grading the quality of evidence and the strength of recommendations I: critical appraisal of existing approaches the GRADE working group. BMC Health Serv Res 2004;4:38.
37. Available at: http://www.gradeworkinggroup.org/. Accessed July 10, 2020.
38. Siu AL, U.S. Preventive Services Task Force. Screening for breast cancer: U.S. preventive services task force recommendation statement. Ann Intern Med 2016;164:279–96.
39. Oeffinger KC, Fontham ET, Etzioni R, et al. Breast cancer screening for women at average risk: 2015 guideline update from the American cancer society. JAMA 2015;314:1599–614.
40. Shekelle P, Eccles MP, Grimshaw JM, et al. When should clinical guidelines be updated? BMJ 2001;323:155–7.
41. Jue JJ, Cunningham S, Lohr K, et al. Developing and testing the agency for healthcare research and quality's national guideline clearinghouse extent of adherence to trustworthy standards (NEATS) instrument. Ann Intern Med 2019; 170:480–7.
42. ECRI guidelines Trust. ECRI guidelines Trust, 2020. Available at: https://guidelines.ecri.org. Accessed July 24, 2020.
43. Brouwers MC, Kerkvliet K, Spithoff K, et al. The AGREE reporting checklist: a tool to improve reporting of clinical practice guidelines. BMJ 2016;352:i1152.
44. Qaseem A, Lin JS, Mustafa RA, et al. Clinical guidelines committee of the american college of p. screening for breast cancer in average-risk women: a guidance statement from the american college of physicians. Ann Intern Med 2019;170:547–60.
45. Qaseem A, Crandall CJ, Mustafa RA, et al. Clinical guidelines committee of the american college of p. screening for colorectal cancer in asymptomatic average-risk adults: a guidance statement from the american college of physicians. Ann Intern Med 2019;171:643–54.
46. Ransohoff DF, Pignone M, Sox HC. How to decide whether a clinical practice guideline is trustworthy. JAMA 2013;309:139–40.
47. Kung J, Miller RR, Mackowiak PA. Failure of Clinical Practice Guidelines to Meet Institute of Medicine Standards: Two More Decades of Little, If Any, Progress. Arch Intern Med 2012;172(21):1–6.

Increasing Cancer Screening Rates in Primary Care

Richard Wender, MD[a],*, Andrew M.D. Wolf, MD[b]

KEYWORDS

- Cancer screening • Primary care • Primary care clinicians • Population management
- Physician reminders • Patient reminders

KEY POINTS

- A recommendation from a trusted source of primary care is one of the strongest predictors of whether screening does or does not occur.
- In order to achieve the highest possible population-wide screening rates, primary care clinicians must embrace the responsibility to screen their entire enrolled patient population, institute several overarching general approaches to screening, and implement a combination of evidence based interventions.
- The result of following the road map outlined in this review is that more patients will be screened, more cancers prevented, and fewer preventable cancer deaths will occur.

Screening for cervix, colorectal, breast and prostate cancer has led to substantial reductions in disease-specific and overall cancer mortality, and screening high-risk populations for lung cancer has been demonstrated to reduce mortality by at least 20%.[1,2] Screening for all of these cancers has been shown to be cost-effective and rank among the most cost-effective of all preventive interventions.[3] In certain scenarios combining screening and treatment, screening for prostate cancer is cost-effective.[4] Achieving high rates of cancer screening, however, is very difficult. Numerous barriers related to how care is organized and delivered in the United States, as well as barriers related to the lives of patients, the neighborhoods they live in, their personal attitudes and beliefs, the availability of primary and specialty care, and financial resources must all be addressed to ensure that the highest possible number of patients derive the proved benefits of cancer screening.[5]

Responsibility for promoting screening varies from country to country. Many high-resource nations that provide some form of national health care centralize the responsibility for recommending and delivering screening services.[6] When done well, high population-wide screening rates are achieved. Primary care clinicians in many of these countries reinforce the recommendation to be screened but are not primarily

[a] Family Medicine and Community Health, Perelman School of Medicine, University of Pennsylvania, Andrew Mutch Building, 51 N. 39th Street, Philadelphia, PA 19104, USA; [b] University of Virginia School of Medicine, Box 800744 UVA Health System, Charlottesville, VA 22908, USA
* Corresponding author.
E-mail address: richard.wender@jefferson.edu

Med Clin N Am 104 (2020) 971–987
https://doi.org/10.1016/j.mcna.2020.08.001
0025-7125/20/© 2020 Elsevier Inc. All rights reserved.

responsible for implementing screening. In the United States, although numerous parts of the health system contribute to screening, responsibility to deliver cancer screening services falls principally on primary care clinicians. For most patients whether or not their primary care clinician recommends that they be screened for a particular cancer is a determining factor in whether screening occurs.[7,8] This article focuses on the role of primary care clinicians and primary care–based systems in achieving the highest possible screening rates for the populations they serve and provides a roadmap for primary care clinicians and their teams to increase screening within their practices.

On a personal note, the authors of this article are all primary care physicians with many combined years dedicated to clinical and public health practice. We know how easy it is to be caught up in the day-to-day rhythms of acute and chronic care management while addressing the multitude of demands on time, resources, and attention. But cancer is the leading cause of death before age 85 years and the leading cause of premature mortality in our nation. Cancer screening will prevent more premature deaths than almost anything else we do in our practices. Failing to achieve the highest possible rates of cancer screening is very costly as measured by avoidable advanced cancer diagnoses and cancer-related death. Mobilizing our clinical teams to help all patients in every community overcome barriers to cancer screening represents one of our best opportunities to reduce the devastating impact of cancer for all.

BARRIERS TO SCREENING

Numerous barriers must be addressed and overcome to increase screening rates. A brief summary of these barriers follows.

Health System Barriers

Individuals who are uninsured and/or do not have access to a primary care clinician are far less likely to be up to date with cancer screening than patients who have health insurance and a trusted source of primary care.[9,10] Usually, but not invariably, patients enrolled in fully integrated health systems that combine a closed network of clinicians with health insurance are more likely to receive screening recommendations and reminders and to be up to date with screening than patients covered by traditional open network health insurance.[11] Aspects of practice organization, particularly practice autonomy and level of support services, correlate with higher screening rates.[12]

Patient-Related Barriers

Although insurance status is a predominant barrier to screening, other patient-related characteristics affect screening. Patients with lower income, lower educational achievement, and less social support are less likely to be up to date with cancer screening. Regardless of income and insurance status, individuals who are less interested in preventive care, actively resistant to screening for cancer, or who must prioritize issues other than health care are less likely to be screened. Cultural factors, language barriers, and certain beliefs, such as nihilism and fatalism, correlate with lower likelihood of being screened.[13] In general, African American, Asian, Hispanic, and Native American/Alaska Native populations are more frequently affected by most of the barriers outlined earlier, which likely contributes to the lower prevalence of screening in these groups compared with other populations.[2,14]

Practice Barriers

Health system and patient-related barriers are intimately tied to the type, number, and complexity of obstacles that a particular primary care practice must overcome to screen all patients. Federally qualified health centers, (FQHCs) and other practices predominately caring for low-income, nonmajority, uninsured, or Medicaid insured populations will find it far more difficult to reach high practice-wide screening rates than practices predominately providing care for a Medicare and commercially insured, higher income population. For example, only 44% of patients cared for in our nation's FQHC's are up to date with colorectal cancer screening compared with the national rate of 68.8%.[15,16] Regardless of the challenges that a practice must identify and overcome, no primary care practice can reach the highest possible screening rates without a deliberate, comprehensive, evidence-informed, sustained practice-wide plan and commitment to screen every eligible patient enrolled in the practice. This invariably requires leadership, practice champions, and commitment to do whatever is necessary to reach everyone, including commitment to address the barriers that must be overcome.

GENERAL PRINCIPLES OF SCREENING

Every practice should be committed to improving practice-wide screening rates. Several fundamental steps must be followed, and specific capacities must be available to guide quality improvement. This section reviews foundational elements required to improve screening, followed by discussion of specific evidence-based interventions.

A Practice-Wide Screening Policy

Every practice must precisely identify and define their cancer screening goals: what diseases will be screened for; who will be screened, including age to start and stop screening; what tests will be used; and if a shared decision-making process will be used.[17] These decisions should be in accord with evidence-based cancer screening guidelines. Constructing high-quality cancer screening guidelines is a complex, expensive, time-consuming process requiring an independent evidence review, an expert, independent guideline authorship panel, and external feedback and review. No practice can reproduce this process on their own. All practices should rely on expert guidelines.

Although numerous organizations develop cancer screening guidelines, the guidelines written by the American Cancer Society and the United States Preventive Services Task Force are the most widely known, respected, and influential.[18] Both groups follow the process described by the National Academy of Science for how to write trustworthy guidelines.[19] The recommendations by the USPSTF and ACS are very similar but not identical (**Table 1**).[20,21] The Affordable Care Act requires that most commercial plans cover all costs of cancer screening tests that receive an A or B rating from the USPSTF.[22] Prostate cancer screening is rated as a C; the other 4 receive an A or B rating. Although considering other cancer screening guidelines is reasonable, the guidelines authored by these 2 major groups should form the basis for practice-wide screening policies.

Defining the Population to be Screened

One of the most important advances in primary care–based screening has been the increasing acceptance of responsibility to screen the entire enrolled population associated with the practice. This broad definition of the practice denominator forms the basis of population-based screening. Figuring out the total list of patients for whom the practice is responsible is demanding. Two approaches are commonly used to identify the list of enrolled patients. In some cases, such as closed panel insurance

Table 1
Age to start cancer screening: US Preventive Services Task Force (USPSTF) and American Cancer Society (ACS)

	USPSTF	ACS
Colorectal cancer	Age 50 y	Age 45y
Breast cancer	Universal screening at age 50 y; shared decision-making at 40–49 y	Universal screening at age 45 y; shared decision-making at 40–44 y
Lung cancer	Age 55 y	Age 55 y
Cervical cancer	Age 21 y	Age 25 y
Prostate cancer	Shared decision-making at age 55 y	Shared decision-making at age 50 y

plans or traditionally capitated plans, patients can be assigned to specific clinicians from a total list of patients who are signed up with a practice. For most of the practices, panels are defined by the visit history. For example, enrolled patients for whom the practice assumes responsibility may be defined by the group of patients who have made a visit within the past year or 2 visits anytime in the previous 2 years. In any case, the practice must be able to define the list of patients and the screening status of each of those patients.

The practice-wide screening rate is determined by measuring the percent of all patients enrolled in the practice who are eligible for screening and who are up to date with the recommended screening test option. (For colorectal cancer and cervical cancer, patients need to be up to date with one of the screening tests from a menu of options.)

Measurement

All quality improvement is predicated on the ability and commitment to measure and report outcomes. In the case of cancer screening, the practice must be able to measure and report practice-wide screening rates and rates for each clinician and generate lists of patients who are not up to date. It is often useful to also identify patients who have never been screened for a particular cancer because these individuals are at particularly high risk for presenting with advanced disease.

Electronic Health Records as Quality Improvement Tools

When the quality "movement" first began, some practices developed stand-alone registries to track screening results. Today, more than 90% of primary care practices use electronic medical records, and almost every practice relies on the electronic health record (EHR) to serve as their quality measurement tool.[23] EHRs have become one of the most important quality improvement aids in all of health care and certainly in primary care. At a minimum, EHRs must function as a registry for all quality initiatives, but the modern-day EHR should do much more. Ideal attributes of a high-functioning EHR in support of cancer screening are listed in **Box 1**.[24]

Mobilizing the Whole Clinical Team

A hallmark of primary care–based quality improvement efforts is a deliberate effort to mobilize the entire clinical team to achieve quality outcomes. Even highly motivated clinicians who strive to recommend screening at every available opportunity cannot,

> **Box 1**
> **Ideal electronic health record attributes in support of cancer screening**
>
> Data gathering
>   Family history, including generating a genogram
>   Past medical history
>   Personal habits, such as tobacco use and alcohol
>   Exposures that affect cancer risk, such as occupational and environmental exposures
>   Cancer screening history, including tests performed, dates, and results
>
> Generate reminders
>   Produce effective, automated reminders at the time of visits
>   Produce patient reminders
>
> Manage population health
>   Generate lists of individuals up to date with screening with contact information
>   Determine practice-wide screening rates and screening rates for each clinician's panel

on their own, overcome a multitude of screening barriers. Models of team-based care are the patient-centered medical home (PCMH)[25] and advanced primary care (APC).[26] Practices earning designation by the National Committee for Quality Assurance (NCQA) such as a PCMH achieve, on average, higher levels of screening for cervical, breast, and colorectal cancers.[27] Specific potential roles for team members include identification of screening status; instituting prompts, reminders, or placing a test order to be signed by the clinician; managing patient outreach and reminders; educating patients about how to complete screening tests; tracking results and generating prompts for tests that are not completed; and facilitating follow-up for those who test positive on initial testing. These varied roles can be met by different categories of team members. Some practices employ screening navigators who can address many of these functions and often play an enhanced role in working directly with patients to overcome unique obstacles that may be rendering their participation more difficult. Greater attention to the role of navigation and navigators follows.

Recommending Screening at Every Visit

A screening recommendation by one's personal source of primary care during a patient visit is a highly effective intervention; patients who receive a recommendation are far more likely to participate in screening than those who do not.[28–30] This recommendation must be delivered clearly and with conviction; patients should not perceive the recommendation as just an option to consider. Preventive care visits, often referred to as wellness visits, present particularly good opportunities to recommend and arrange cancer screening.[31] Screening recommended during a visit for this, or any other purpose, such as for acute care or chronic disease management, is often called opportunistic screening. Incorporating screening into both visit categories must be a priority for all primary care practices and all clinicians. Although relying only on recommendations to screen given during visits is not a sufficient strategy to achieve the highest possible rates, these recommendations are crucial and can result in reasonably high screening rates. Every practice should strive to ensure that eligible individuals receive age- and risk-appropriate screening recommendations during all visits, regardless of the purpose of the visit. Striving to recommend cancer screening at every opportunity, although almost impossible to perfectly achieve, represents a vital opportunity to increase screening.

Wellness Visits

A series of studies found the concept of the annual check-up to be ineffective.[32] This research resulted in gradual abandonment of the annual check-up and a period where the role of some form of regular visit dedicated to wellness or prevention was abandoned. These findings, however, were counterbalanced by a series of studies revolving around the value of preventive visits to increase cancer screening rates.[33] These findings have gradually catalyzed a redefinition of preventive care visits, culminating in CMS's creation of an annual Wellness benefit as a part of the Affordable Care Act.[34] Many insurance companies now encourage their enrollees to have wellness visits and provide incentives to clinicians to conduct these visits.

Unlike the annual check-up from decades ago, which did not include crisply defined elements linked to evidence-based guidelines, the modern-day annual wellness visit usually specifies a minimal set of elements that must be included in order to meet requirements for billing. These elements are usually derived from evidence-based guidelines. Adoption of wellness visits varies substantially, and use of the Medicare annual wellness visit benefit has been low.[35] Although the highly prescriptive nature of the wellness visit requirements help ensure that important services are provided at the visit, this model also creates an administrative burden for practices. In fact, fulfilling the visit requirements demands a coordinated team-based approach; many practices do not have the infrastructure or have not created the processes to smoothly deliver wellness visits.

Opportunistic Screening

Administering vaccines to children at every opportunity, including visits for acute concerns, has become a care standard.[36] This approach is supported by use of immunization registries and standing practice-wide orders. A similar approach can be taken to preventive care for adults; recommending cancer screening to those due for screening as a part of sick visits or visits for chronic disease management represents a crucial strategy to maximize screening rates. Incorporating screening into as many visits as possible is a proven and necessary strategy.

In order to achieve the aspirational goal of recommending screening at every visit, practices must implement team-based solutions to overcome impediments to screening. Obstacles to opportunistic screening must be systematically addressed. These obstacles include short duration of visits and competing agenda, including addressing patient concerns, managing disease, and implementing other aspects of preventive care, yet can be overcome by such strategies as delegating nonphysician personnel to implement cancer screening tests via standing orders. Variable capacities of EHRs to facilitate screening may enhance or impede opportunistic screening.

INTERVENTIONS TO INCREASE CANCER SCREENING

In addition to cancer screening policies, standing orders, mobilization of the clinical team, and screening at every visit, several practice-based interventions directed at the clinical team function have been proved to increase screening rates. These are summarized in **Boxes 2** and **3**.

Financial Incentives and New Payment Models

Over the past 15 years, increasing emphasis has been placed on the provision of high-quality care. Emerging innovative risk-based payment models and new Medicare payment systems provide variable reimbursement for services based on level of quality achieved. As outlined in the Medicare Access and CHIP Reauthorization Act of 2015 (MACRA), CMS is now transitioning to the Quality Payment Program. This program rewards high-quality care through 2 mechanisms: Advanced Alternative Payment Models and the Merit-based Incentive Payment System (MIPS). The most

---

Box 2
Fundamental requirements to increase cancer screening in primary care

1. Commitment to increase cancer screening rates

2. A clearly defined screening policy—based on well-established cancer screening guidelines

3. Reliance on a high-performing electronic health record

4. Screening at every visit

5. Encouraging wellness visits

6. Embracing population management

---

important element in the MIPS program is level of achievement in evidence-based quality measures. Several cancer screening measures are included in essentially all quality-based payment models. Linking quality and payment has led to profound changes in the organization of primary care practice. Many practices have instituted steps to improve quality, have sought training, hired additional staff, instituted measurement, and learned how to incorporate quality improvement into routine practice. MACRA is designed to give practical options for small practices to allow them to participate. Failure to participate places limits on the reimbursements practices are eligible to receive.[37]

Payment for quality has been instituted inconsistently throughout the country. For some clinicians in some systems, "pay for performance" has become an important influence, a true paradigm shift. For payment and incentives to effectively promote practice, dollars at stake should be substantial, either contributing to higher reimbursement through attainment of high-quality or avoiding payment penalties for the failure to achieve quality milestones. Interestingly, penalty avoidance has been shown to be a somewhat more effective way to affect practice than a positive incentive.[38]

Continuous Quality Improvement

The most commonly used model of continuous quality improvement (CQI) is called rapid cycle improvement, and the most common specific procedure is called Plan-Do-Study-Act (PDSA). PDSA cycles encourage practices to come up with a plan, execute throughout the practice or in part of the practice, measure the effect of the

---

Box 3
Primary care interventions proved to increase cancer screening

1. Financial incentives and new payment models

2. Continuous quality improvement

3. Clinician reminders

4. Audit and feedback

5. Patient reminders or prompts

6. Population management

7. Screening navigation

8. Combining multiple interventions

---

intervention, and then either spread the intervention to the entire practice, continue the intervention, or alter it to try something else. The PDSA model discourages inaction and overstudy. Regardless of the model used, primary care practices are encouraged to be consistently engaged in the process of improving quality of care. One systematic review of the effects of implementing CQI and PDSA revealed definite but small improvements in care. Failure to achieve greater progress seemed to relate, in part, to incomplete implementation of the model.[39]

Population Management

One of the most important advances in clinical quality improvement related to prevention and chronic disease management has been the integration of population management methodology into primary care practices and broader health care systems. Population management is a general term referring to a set of activities that occur outside of clinical encounters designed both to capture important characteristics and clinical milestones for all patients enrolled in a system or individual practice, as well as to implement interventions that encourage and help patients receive preventive care, often without requiring an office visit.[40]

True population management demands that the system or practice has ways to reach out to individual patients outside of clinical encounters to encourage them to alter their behavior, come in for care, or to get a test. Most cancer screening population management studies are theory based and evaluate various ways to contact and prompt patients to participate in cancer screening. The most commonly evaluated methods of outreach are by letter, phone call, or, more recently, text. In some cases, reminders are tailored to take advantage of patient preference for a particular approach to screening where more than one screening test can be chosen. The relative efficacy of these different types of interventions varies depending on the population being studied. In general, all types of reminders can increase participation in cancer screening. Phone reminders, with or without tailoring, are usually found to be more effective than mailed interventions.[41,42] On the other hand, some systems that have long-standing, mature mailed patient reminder programs have achieved very high colorectal screening adherence.[43,44]

Quality Measures—A Two-Edged Sword

Although linking quality care to payment can change clinician and health system behavior, pay for performance can promote screening for some cancers and simultaneously reduce the emphasis on screening for others. Although screening, with or without a shared decision, is recommended for 5 different cancers, quality measures exist only for colorectal cancer, cervix cancer, and breast cancer—but only for women older than 50 years. In the absence of a quality measure, less than 15% of eligible individuals have been screened for lung cancer, and prostate cancer screening has declined significantly in the past decade.[45] Unlike the situation for the other cancers, the relevant metric for prostate cancer screening should be proportion of patients offered shared decision-making, rather than proportion actually screened, because prostate screening guidelines call for shared decision-making rather than routine screening.

Clinician Reminders

Reminders directed at primary care providers (PCPs) to improve cancer screening rates have been in use for many years and have evolved with the increasing sophistication of record keeping technology and increasing array of screening options used for cancer early detection and prevention. Paper flowcharts filled in by hand and handwritten tickler files have largely transitioned to EHR-generated automated reminders with integrated decision support and test ordering. Provider reminders have been consistently identified as one of the key provider-centered facilitators to promote cancer screening. Conversely, lack of a reminder or tracking system has been cited as a provider-centered barrier to screening, along with lack of time, forgetfulness, acute care visits, patient comorbidities, and patient refusal.[46–48] Before the advent of EHRs, use of reminder systems was sporadic. In a 1990 survey of community-based primary care physicians, only a quarter were using any formal mechanism to promote cancer screening, with only 17% reporting use of a reminder system.[49] Although EHRs generally include some type of reminder capability, their utilization is far from universal. In a 2014 national survey, only 49% of PCPs reported availability of EHR support for breast cancer screening and 46% for cervical cancer screening. Designation as a PCMH was associated with a greater likelihood of having a system in place. As recently as 2016, only 45% of FQHCs reported using provider reminder systems.[50] In a 2015 survey of Indian Health Service Tribal facilities, only 65% were using a health care provider reminder system for colorectal cancer (CRC) screening.[51]

Manual, computer-generated, and EHR-embedded reminder systems are all in use, and all of them have been shown in well-controlled studies to be effective, although resulting improvements in cancer screening rates vary based on practice setting and cancer test. A 2019 Cochrane review determined with moderate certainty that manually generated paper reminders improve physician adherence to cancer screening with a median improvement of 8.5% over usual care.[52] A 2017 Cochrane review of computer-generated reminders delivered on paper found that such interventions "probably slightly" improve provider adherence to preventive guidelines, although the review was not limited to cancer screening. The median improvement was 6.8%.[53]

The Veteran's Administration (VA) conducted a retrospective descriptive cohort study examining the impact of activating an electronic reminder linked to an option to order lung cancer screening for 9170 patients in the VA system. Of those opting in, 76% completed screening during the 6-month study period, although the baseline rate was not reported.[54] In a cluster-randomized trial of an EHR prompt for CRC screening, there was no increase in screening based on the intention-to-screen analysis but there was somewhat more screening in the per-protocol analysis. Patients in both arms of the study had been invited to participate in fecal immunochemical (FIT) testing, which may have diluted the impact of the EHR intervention.[55] An "active choice" EHR intervention giving PCPs the option to order or cancel colonoscopy and/or mammography for overdue patients during office visits demonstrated a 12% increase in orders for both tests compared with control practices. Screening completion rates were significantly greater for colonoscopies but not for mammography.[56]

Of importance, many investigators have conducted studies of reminder systems in practices caring for low socioeconomic and minority populations. Although the magnitude of the impact varies depending on the number and intensity of interventions included, reminder systems are generally found to be very effective in practices serving these communities. Another way to look at these data is that usual care is often woefully inadequate to promote screening. Some practices can achieve remarkable increases in screening rates by using reminders with or without other interventions.[57–59]

Audit and Feedback

One method of promoting population management is to use data from the EHR to both report screening rates for the panels managed by individual clinicians and to provide the clinician with lists of patients who are overdue for screening. Two systematic reviews found that provider audit and feedback is linked to improved screening rates for breast and cervical cancer and for fecal occult blood (FOBT) CRC screening. There was insufficient evidence for colonoscopy.[60,61] More recently, a cluster-randomized trial of providing lists of patients due for FOBT screening to PCPs every 4 months for a year led to slightly greater screening rates in the intervention arm (32.9% vs 31.2%).[62] In a practice-level controlled study in which PCPs received rosters of patients due for CRC screening linked to the option of either a reminder letter or outreach by a delegate, test ordering was significantly higher in the intervention practices (88% vs 80.5%), as was screening completion (81 vs 78%).[63] The small absolute improvement was likely due to the very high baseline screening rate in these academic practices. In a setting with much lower baseline screening rates, a similar CRC screening intervention had a much greater impact; PCPs in the intervention practices received lists of overdue patients and were prompted to either see, telephone, or email their patients. The outreach could be conducted by either PCPs or assistants. The CRC screening completion rate was 33.5% among intervention patients, compared with 19% in the control arm. Of note, there was no difference based on PCP or assistant contact, supporting the effectiveness of involving nonphysicians in the screening process.

Patient Outreach and Reminders

One aspect of population management is to conduct various forms of outreach to patients who are due for cancer screening. Outreach can also be referred to as patient reminders. Outreach can take a variety of forms, ranging from mailed outreach, phone calls, or texts. In the case of colorectal cancer screening, mailings can include FIT tests as well. Outreach messages can be general or tailored. Tailoring can be based on expressed patient preferences and/or evidence of culturally appropriate messages proved to be motivating. Numerous studies of patient outreach have been conducted, and evidence of effectiveness is incontrovertible, although the magnitude of the intervention effect varies between cancer screens being targeted and between specific interventions. For colorectal cancer, patient reminders alone can increase screening rates by about 20%.[64] A review of text reminders reports increases in screening from 0.6% to 15% for several cancers.[65] A systematic review of a range of CRC screening interventions found that pre-FIT and post-FIT reminders demonstrated modest efficacy with median 4.1% and 3.1% improvement in CRC screening, respectively. The review also found that mailed FIT outreach was consistently effective with a median improvement in CRC screening of 21.5% across the 10 studies evaluating this intervention.[66] Other investigators have reported variable benefit, with mailed FIT outreach depending on how the program is designed and executed.[67,68]

Comparative Effectiveness of Strategies to Improve Cancer Screening Rates

Primary care practices may need to choose how to start a quality improvement project to increase screening. A systematic review from 2001 examined physician reminders, mailed patient reminders, or combined physician-patient strategies to increase breast and cervical cancer screening. It found that patient-based strategies increased screening rates by 10% overall; physician-based strategies increased screening by 6% to 40%; and combined strategies increased screening by 5% to 35%. The investigators concluded that the most effective strategies were physician-based strategies and that computerized and manual reminders were more effective than audits with feedback.[69] A 2002 meta-analysis included 108 trials evaluating strategies to improve mammography, cervical, and CRC screening rates and calculated odds ratios (OR) for effectiveness compared with usual care. The strategies, in descending order of effectiveness, included organizational change (OR 2.5–17.6); patient financial incentives (OR 1.8–2.8); patient reminders (OR 1.7–2.75); provider education (OR 1.7–3.0); provider reminders (OR 1.4–1.7); patient education (OR1.3–1.4); and provider feedback (OR 1.1–1.8).[70]

Screening Navigation

Most of the interventions reviewed here only modestly increase screening rates, and none are sufficient to achieve the highest level of screening possible. Using screening navigators who take responsibility for many of the interventions described here has been demonstrated to help overcome even the most daunting barriers to screening.[71–75] The defining aspect of screening navigation is that team members in the practice are specifically trained to promote cancer screening. Practices may hire individuals who exclusively serve as navigators or may carve out time for existing team members to work as navigators. Navigators may be assigned to help organize management of chronic diseases, such as diabetes, in addition to screening navigation.

Screening navigation increases screening rates, and the incremental increase in rates is greatest in individuals facing the greatest barriers to screening. A study by Percac-Lima and colleagues in community health centers focused on patients facing multiple barriers, including poverty and language challenges, found that 10.2% of patients randomized to receive navigation services were up to date for all recommended cancer screens compared with 6.8% of control patients. Effect size for individual cancers was higher, with the intervention group being from 6% to 8% more likely to be up to date for each individual cancer, including screening for breast cancer, colorectal cancer, or cervical cancer.[76] A CRC screening navigation program in rural Georgia found a 4-fold increase in CRC screening among navigated patients compared with controls (43% vs 11%).[77]

The primary challenge confronting practices that want to institute screening navigation is being able to afford the service. The National Colorectal Cancer Roundtable produced a tool addressing this important issue providing specific suggestions on how to afford navigation. Specific strategies include demonstrating value to health systems, insurers, and employers; participating in pay for performance contracts; seeking grants; and using creative new staffing models.[78]

Combining Interventions

One of the consistent findings across all studies of quality improvement to increase screening rates is that single interventions only modestly increase screening rates. Almost invariably, combining multiple interventions is required to achieve very high rates. Overall, studies suggest that the greater the number of interventions, the greater the impact on cancer screening rates. In a Canadian PCP survey linked to CRC screening rates, for example, practices that reported using 4 to 5 strategies had rates 27% higher than those reporting using 0 to 1 strategy.[79] Most multicomponent interventions have yielded greater improvements in screening rates than has been reported for PCP reminders alone. At the low end of effectiveness, an intervention using a before-after design that incorporated pay-for-performance incentives and patient and provider reminders yielded a 5% increase in mammography rates and a 6% increase in Pap tests, both statistically significant.[80] At the other end of the spectrum, interventions involving patient reminder letters, provider education, patient education, and/or practice workflow alterations, along with PCP reminders, have yielded screening rate increases of 32% to 37%.[81]

A ROADMAP TO INCREASING SCREENING RATES

Every adult primary care practice and every health system that provides primary care services is obligated to achieve the highest cancer screening rates possible. Failure to invest in the people and interventions required to overcome the numerous barriers to cancer screening will inevitably result in excess incidence of preventable cancers and avoidable cancer mortality. Along with continuing to reduce rates of tobacco use, increasing evidence-based cancer screening defines the nation's best opportunity to reduce suffering and death from cancer. Systems should follow these 10 steps to improving screening rates.

1. Count on leaders and champions: leaders of the system and/or individual practices should unambiguously endorse the value of cancer screening and set it as a major priority. A champion or champions should be identified who can spearhead a coordinated effort to increasing rates.
2. Measure progress and report regularly: utilizing the practice EHR, a system to easily measure and report screening rates for all 5 recommended cancers for which screening is recommended, should be developed. Screening rates should become part of the quality dashboard and reported regularly, preferably monthly, to the entire practice.
3. Harness the EHR capacity: many modern day EHRs have the capacity to support many of the steps necessary to support screening. EHR manufacturers have the obligation to include these elements at no additional cost or, at least, at minimal cost. Practices need to use the full scope of supportive features, from risk assessment, to reminders, to measurement, and to population management to maximize screening rates.
4. Create empowered teams with defined roles: everyone in the practice should be accountable for achieving the outcome of higher screening rates.
5. Screen at every visit: although wellness visits are particularly good opportunities to promote screening, too few patients participate in preventive visits. Recommend cancer screening at every opportunity.
6. Implement multiple interventions: a large array of interventions increase screening rates, but no one intervention is likely to be sufficient. Combine multiple interventions.
7. Measure the effect of every step: use the Plan-Do-Study-Act model to continuously work to push screening rates higher.
8. Manage the whole population: many patients do not come in to the office regularly. Institute population outreach.
9. Find a way to provide screening navigation: Screening navigators help overcome the most difficult barriers to screening.
10. Celebrate success: whether or not the practice has a financial incentive to improve screening, success should be widely shared and celebrated as a team.

Increasing cancer screening is very hard work but few interventions in all of primary care prevent more deaths. In the United States, what does or does not occur in the primary care setting is a major determinant of the screening rates we achieve. Evidence-based interventions illuminate the pathway to higher screening rates.

REFERENCES

1. Siegel RL, Miller KD, Jemal A. Cancer statistics, 2020. CA Cancer J Clin 2020; 70(1):7–30.

2. Smith RA, Andrews KS, Brooks D, et al. Cancer screening in the United States, 2019: A review of current American Cancer Society guidelines and current issues in cancer screening. CA Cancer J Clin 2019;69(3):184–210.

3. Maciosek MV, LaFrance AB, Dehmer SP, et al. Updated Priorities Among Effective Clinical Preventive Services. Ann Fam Med 2017;15(1):14–22.

4. de Carvalho TM, Heijnsdijk EAM, de Koning HJ, et al. Comparative effectiveness of prostate cancer screening between the ages of 55 and 69 years followed by active surveillance. Cancer 2018;124:507.

5. Wender RC, Brawley OW, Fedewa SA, et al. A blueprint for cancer screening and early detection: Advancing screening's contribution to cancer control. CA Cancer J Clin 2019;69(1):50–79.

6. Basu P, Ponti A, Anttila A, et al. Status of implementation and organization of cancer screening in The European Union Member States-Summary results from the second European screening report. Int J Cancer 2018;142(1):44–56 [published correction appears in Int J Cancer. 2018;143(1):E1].

7. Crabtree BF, Miller WL, Tallia AF, et al. Delivery of clinical preventive services in family medicine offices. Ann Fam Med 2005;3:430–5.

8. Brawarsky P, Brooks DR, Mucci LA, et al. Effect of physician recommendation and patient adherence on rates of colorectal cancer testing. Cancer Detect Prev 2004;28(4):260–8.

9. Hall IJ, Tangka FKL, Sabatino SA, et al. Patterns and Trends in Cancer Screening in the United States. Prev Chronic Dis 2018;15:E97.

10. Toyoda Y, Oh EJ, Premaratne ID, et al. Affordable Care Act State-Specific Medicaid Expansion: Impact on Health Insurance Coverage and Breast Cancer Screening Rate. J Am Coll Surg 2020. https://doi.org/10.1016/j.jamcollsurg. 2020.01.031.

11. Levin TR, Jamieson L, Burley DA, et al. Organized colorectal cancer screening in integrated health care systems. Epidemiol Rev 2011;33:101–10.

12. Elizabeth MY, Lynn MS, Patricia HP, et al. Primary Care Practice Organization Influences Colorectal Cancer Screening Performance. Health Res Educ Trust 2007. https://doi.org/10.1111/j.1475-6773.2006.00643.x.

13. Ely JW, Levy BT, Daly J, et al. Patient Beliefs About Colon Cancer Screening. J Cancer Educ 2016;31(1):39–46.

14. Nagelhout E, Comarell K, Samadder NJ, et al. Barriers to Colorectal Cancer Screening in a Racially Diverse Population Served by a Safety-Net Clinic. J Community Health 2017;42(4):791–6.

15. Available at: https://www.cdc.gov/cancer/colorectal/statistics/use-screening-tests-BRFSS.htm.

16. Available at: https://nccrt.org/wp-content/uploads/Nguyen-CRC-MNguyen-NCCRT.pdf.

17. Sarfaty M, Wender R. How to Increase Colorectal Cancer Screening Rates in Practice. CA Cancer J Clin 2007;57 Nov-Dec:354–66.

18. Kwon HT, Ma GX, Gold RS, et al. Primary care physicians' cancer screening recommendation practices and perceptions of cancer risk of Asian Americans. Asian Pac J Cancer Prev 2013;14(3):1999–2004.

19. Institute of Medicine (US) Committee on Standards for Developing Trustworthy Clinical Practice Guidelines. In: Graham R, Mancher M, Miller Wolman D, et al, editors. Clinical practice guidelines we can trust. Washington (DC): National Academies Press (US); 2011. Available at: https://www.ncbi.nlm.nih.gov/books/NBK209539/.

20. Available at: https://www.uspreventiveservicestaskforce.org/uspstf/recommendation/colorectal-cancer-screening. Accessed September 29, 2020.

21. Wolf AMD, Fontham ETH, Church TR, et al. Colorectal cancer screening for average-risk adults: 2018 guideline update from the American Cancer Society. CA Cancer J Clin 2018;68(4):250-81. doi: 10.3322/caac.21457. Epub 2018 May 30. PMID: 29846947.

22. Chait N, Glied S. Promoting Prevention Under the Affordable Care Act. Annu Rev Public Health 2018;39:507–24.

23. Available at: https://dashboard.healthit.gov/quickstats/quickstats.php#:%7E:text=As%20of%20January%202016%2C%20over,certified%20EHR%20technology%20(CEHRT).

24. Available at: https://www.ehrinpractice.com/ehr-features-guide.html.

25. Sarfaty M, Wender R, Smith R. Promoting cancer screening within the patient centered medical home. CA Cancer J Clin 2011;61(6):397–408.

26. Bazemore A, Neale AV, Lupo P, et al. Advancing the Science of Implementation in Primary Health Care. J Am Board Fam Med 2018;31(3):307–11.

27. Available at: https://www.ncqa.org/wp-content/uploads/2019/09/20190926_PCMH_Evidence_Report.pdf.

28. Harry ML, Truitt AR, Saman DM, et al. Barriers and facilitators to implementing cancer prevention clinical decision support in primary care: a qualitative study. BMC Health Serv Res 2019;19(1):534.

29. Patel K, Gishe J, Liu J, et al. Factors Influencing Recommended Cancer Screening in Low-Income African American Women in Tennessee. J Racial Ethn Health Disparities 2020;7(1):129–36.

30. Honein-AbouHaidar GN, Kastner M, Vuong V, et al. Systematic Review and Meta-study Synthesis of Qualitative Studies Evaluating Facilitators and Barriers to Participation in Colorectal Cancer Screening. Cancer Epidemiol Biomarkers Prev 2016;25(6):907–17.

31. Fenton JJ, Cai Y, Weiss NS, et al. Delivery of cancer screening: how important is the preventive health examination? Arch Intern Med 2007;167:580–5.

32. Krogsbøll LT, Jørgensen KJ, Gøtzsche PC. General health checks in adults for reducing morbidity and mortality from disease. Cochrane Database Syst Rev 2019;(1):CD009009.

33. Simpson VL, Kovich M. Outcomes of primary care-based Medicare annual wellness visits with older adults: A scoping review. Geriatr Nurs 2019;40(6):590–6.

34. Beckman AL, Becerra AZ, Marcus A, et al. Medicare Annual Wellness Visit association with healthcare quality and costs. Am J Manag Care 2019;25(3):e76–82.

35. Bluestein D, Diduk-Smith R, Jordan L, et al. Medicare Annual Wellness Visits: How to Get Patients and Physicians on Board. Fam Pract Manag 2017;24(2):12–6.

36. Mirza A, Rathore MH. Immunization Update V. Adv Pediatr 2015;62(1):11–27.

37. Miller P, Mosley K. Physician Reimbursement: From Fee-for-Service to MACRA, MIPS and Knudsen SV, Laursen HVB, Johnsen SP, Bartels PD, Ehlers LH, Mainz J. Can quality. J Med Pract Manage 2016;31(5):266–9.

38. Emanuel EJ, Ubel PA, Kessler JB, et al. Using behavioral economics to design physician incentives that deliver high-value care. Ann Intern Med 2016;164(2):114–9.

39. Can continuous quality improvement improve the quality of care? A systematic review of reported effects and methodological rigor in plan-do-study-act projects. BMC Health Serv Res 2019;19(1):683.

40. Kamstra B, Huntington MK. Population Health Management and Cancer Screening. S D Med 2017;(Spec No):37–41.
41. Ritvo PG, Myers RE, Paszat LF, et al. Personal navigation increases colorectal cancer screening uptake. Cancer Epidemiol Biomarkers Prev 2015;24(3):506–11.
42. Myers RE, Sifri R, Daskalakis C, et al. Increasing colon cancer screening in primary care among African Americans. J Natl Cancer Inst 2014;106(12):dju344.
43. Levin TR, Corley DA, Jensen CD, et al. Effects of Organized Colorectal Cancer Screening on Cancer Incidence and Mortality in a Large Community-Based Population. Gastroenterology 2018;155(5):1383–91.e5.
44. Long MD, Lance T, Robertson D, et al. Colorectal Cancer Testing in the National Veterans Health Administration. Dig Dis Sci 2012;57(2):288–93.
45. Yong PC, Sigel K, Rehmani S, et al. Lung Cancer Screening Uptake in the United States. Chest 2020;157(1):236–8.
46. Wender RC. Barriers to screening for colorectal cancer. Gastrointest Endosc Clin N Am 2002;12(1):145–70.
47. Wender RC. Cancer screening and prevention in primary care. Obstacles for physicians. Cancer 1993;72(3 Suppl):1093–9.
48. Lei F, Lee E. Barriers to Lung Cancer Screening With Low-Dose Computed Tomography. Oncol Nurs Forum 2019;46(2):E60–71.
49. Selinger HA, Gregorio DI, Strelez LA. Practices around periodic cancer screening by physicians in primary care specialties. Conn Med 1991;55(8):443–8.
50. Schapira MM, Sprague BL, Klabunde CN, et al. Inadequate systems to support breast and cervical cancer screening in primary care practice. J Gen Intern Med 2016;31(10):1148–55.
51. Available at: https://www.ihs.gov/sites/provider/themes/responsive2017/display_objects/documents/2010_2019/PROV0215.pdf.
52. Arditi C, Rège-Walther M, Durieux P, et al. Computer-generated reminders delivered on paper to healthcare professionals: effects on professional practice and healthcare outcomes. Cochrane Database Syst Rev 2017;(7):CD001175.
53. Pantoja T, Grimshaw JM, Colomer N, et al. Manually-generated reminders delivered on paper: effects on professional practice and patient outcomes. Cochrane Database Syst Rev 2019;(12):CD001174.
54. Federman DG, Kravetz JD, Lerz KA, et al. Implementation of an electronic clinical reminder to improve rates of lung cancer screening. Am J Med 2014;127(9):813–6.
55. Guiriguet C, Muñoz-Ortiz L, Burón A, et al. Alerts in electronic medical records to promote a colorectal cancer screening programme: a cluster randomised controlled trial in primary care. Br J Gen Pract 2016;66(648):e483–90.
56. Patel MS, Volpp KG, Small DS, et al. Using active choice within the electronic health record to increase physician ordering and patient completion of high-value cancer screening tests. Healthc (Amst) 2016;4(4):340–5.
57. Roetzheim RG, Christman LK, Jacobsen PB, et al. A randomized controlled trial to increase cancer screening among attendees of community health centers. Ann Fam Med 2004;2(4):294–300.
58. Otero-Sabogal R, Owens D, Canchola J, et al. Improving rescreening in community clinics: does a system approach work? J Community Health 2006;31(6):497–519.
59. Masi CM, Blackman DJ, Peek ME. Interventions to enhance breast cancer screening, diagnosis, and treatment among racial and ethnic minority women. Med Care Res Rev 2007;64(5 Suppl):195S–242S.

60. Sabatino SA, Lawrence B, Elder R, et al. Effectiveness of interventions to increase screening for breast, cervical, and colorectal cancers: nine updated systematic reviews for the guide to community preventive services. Am J Prev Med 2012; 43(1):97–118.

61. Brouwers MC, De Vito C, Bahirathan L, et al. What implementation interventions increase cancer screening rates? a systematic review. Implement Sci 2011; 6:111.

62. Le Breton J, Ferrat É, Attali C, et al. Effect of reminders mailed to general practitioners on colorectal cancer screening adherence: a cluster-randomized trial. Eur J Cancer Prev 2016;25(5):380–7.

63. Wu CA, Mulder AL, Zai AH, et al. A population management system for improving colorectal cancer screening in a primary care setting. J Eval Clin Pract 2016; 22(3):319–28.

64. Gabrielli E, Bastiampillai AJ, Pontello M, et al. Observational study to evaluate the impact of internet reminders for GPs on colorectal cancer screening uptake in Northern Italy in 2013. J Prev Med Hyg 2016;57(4):E211–5.

65. Dougherty MK, Brenner AT, Crockett SD, et al. Evaluation of Interventions Intended to Increase Colorectal Cancer Screening Rates in the United States: A Systematic Review and Meta-analysis. JAMA Intern Med 2018;178(12):1645–58.

66. Uy C, Lopez J, Trinh-Shevrin C, et al. Text Messaging Interventions on Cancer Screening Rates: A Systematic Review. J Med Internet Res 2017;19(8):e296.

67. Coronado GD, Petrik AF, Vollmer WM, et al. Effectiveness of a Mailed Colorectal Cancer Screening Outreach Program in Community Health Clinics: The STOP CRC Cluster Randomized Clinical Trial. JAMA Intern Med 2018;178(9):1174–81 [published correction appears in JAMA Intern Med. 2019;179(7):1007].

68. Mehta SJ, Pepe RS, Gabler NB, et al. Effect of Financial Incentives on Patient Use of Mailed Colorectal Cancer Screening Tests: A Randomized Clinical Trial. JAMA Netw Open 2019;2(3):e191156 [published correction appears in JAMA Netw Open. 2019 Apr 5;2(4):e193771].

69. Kupets R, Covens A. Strategies for the implementation of cervical and breast cancer screening of women by primary care physicians. Gynecol Oncol 2001; 83(2):186–97.

70. Stone EG, Morton SC, Hulscher ME, et al. Interventions that increase use of adult immunization and cancer screening services: a meta-analysis. Ann Intern Med 2002;136(9):641–51.

71. Shusted CS, Barta JA, Lake M, et al. The Case for Patient Navigation in Lung Cancer Screening in Vulnerable Populations: A Systematic Review. Popul Health Manag 2019;22(4):347–61.

72. Wender R. Cancer Screening Navigation: From Promising Practice to Standard of Care. JAMA Intern Med 2016;176(7):937–8.

73. Sunny A, Rustveld L. The Role of Patient Navigation on Colorectal Cancer Screening Completion and Education: a Review of the Literature. J Cancer Educ 2018;33(2):251–9.

74. Domingo JB, Braun KL. Characteristics of Effective Colorectal Cancer Screening Navigation Programs in Federally Qualified Health Centers: A Systematic Review. J Health Care Poor Underserved 2017;28(1):108–26.

75. Allaire BT, Ekwueme D, Hoerger TJ, et al. Cost-effectiveness of patient navigation for breast cancer screening in the National Breast and Cervical Cancer Early Detection Program. Cancer Causes Control 2019;30(9):923–9.

76. Percac-Lima S, Ashburner JM, Zai AH, et al. Patient Navigation for Comprehensive Cancer Screening in High-Risk Patients Using a Population-Based Health

Information Technology System: A Randomized Clinical Trial. JAMA Intern Med 2016;176(7):930–7.

77. Honeycutt S, Green R, Ballard D, et al. Evaluation of a patient navigation program to promote colorectal cancer screening in rural Georgia, USA. Cancer 2013; 119(16):3059–66.

78. Available at: https://nccrt.org/resource/paying-colorectal-cancer-screening-patient-navigation-toolkit/.

79. Aragones A, Schwartz MD, Shah NR, et al. A randomized controlled trial of a multilevel intervention to increase colorectal cancer screening among Latino immigrants in a primary care facility. J Gen Intern Med 2010;25(6):564–7.

80. Kaczorowski J, Hearps SJ, Lohfeld L, et al. Effect of provider and patient reminders, deployment of nurse practitioners, and financial incentives on cervical and breast cancer screening rates. Can Fam Physician 2013;59(6):e282–9.

81. Hills RL, Kulbok PA, Clark M. Evaluating a Quality Improvement Program for Cervical Cancer Screening at an Urban Safety Net Clinic. Health Promot Pract 2015; 16(5):631–41.

Cancer Screening in Older Adults

Individualized Decision-Making and Communication Strategies

Ashwin A. Kotwal, MD, MS[a,b,*], Louise C. Walter, MD[a,b]

KEYWORDS

- Older adults • Cancer screening • Mammogram • PSA test • Colon cancer
- Lung cancer

KEY POINTS

- The benefits of cancer screening are uncertain in older adults due to lack of inclusion of adults older than 75 in most randomized controlled trials.
- There are several known harms of cancer screening in older adults, including risks of over-diagnosis, false positive results, and procedural complications from downstream diagnostic interventions that increase with decreasing life expectancy.
- Cancer screening recommendations should be individualized for older adults by accounting for overall health and life expectancy, values and preferences, and how these affect specific risks and benefits of cancer screening tests.
- Communicating screening recommendations should incorporate visual data when possible, provide context in terms of competing medical priorities, and use phrases considered more acceptable and easy to understand by older adults.

INTRODUCTION

National recommendations for cancer screening have changed significantly in recent years for older adults.[1] Changes have been related to an increased recognition that cancer screening decisions are often complex in adults who are older than 75 years. Although many older adults have substantial life expectancy and are in good health, most randomized controlled trials (RCTs) of cancer screening tests have not included adults older than 75.[2] Consequently, it can be unclear when it is appropriate to

[a] Division of Geriatrics, Department of Medicine, University of California, San Francisco, San Francisco, CA, USA; [b] Geriatrics, Palliative, and Extended Care Service Line, San Francisco Veterans Affairs Medical Center, San Francisco, CA, USA
* Corresponding author. San Francisco VA, 4150 Clement Street (181G), San Francisco, CA 94121.
E-mail address: ashwin.kotwal@ucsf.edu

Med Clin N Am 104 (2020) 989–1006
https://doi.org/10.1016/j.mcna.2020.08.002
0025-7125/20/© 2020 Elsevier Inc. All rights reserved.
medical.theclinics.com

extrapolate potential benefits to individual older adults seen in clinic. Moreover, there is accumulating evidence of potential harms of cancer screening.[3] For example, older adults who are frail or who have many comorbid medical conditions may experience greater rates of complications from follow-up procedures to screening tests and be unaware of "diagnostic cascades" following positive tests. Overdiagnosis, or the diagnosis and treatment of a cancer that would not have caused symptoms during an individual's remaining lifetime, occurs more frequently among older adults with less than a 10-year life expectancy, potentially exposing them to the harms of testing and treatment (including surgeries, chemotherapy, and radiation) without benefits.[4] Moreover, in typical time-limited primary care settings, discussions about cancer screening may take time away from discussing interventions for treating known comorbid diseases, such as heart disease, or reducing polypharmacy.

In response to the need to balance the potential benefits and harms, cancer screening should not follow the "check-box" approach based solely on age. Rather, cancer screening is a medical procedure that requires thoughtful individualized decision making in older adults before undergoing testing. In practice, however, it can be challenging to communicate cancer screening recommendations while reconciling different, and often inconsistent, cancer screening guidelines. This can lead to both missed opportunities to refer older adults who would benefit from screening, and situations in which screening potentially leads to more harm than benefit. We therefore have 2 objectives in this article. First, we discuss a framework for individualized decision making for prostate, lung, breast, and colon cancer screening. Second, we provide guidance on how to communicate cancer screening recommendations, including recommendations to stop screening when appropriate.

APPROACH TO INDIVIDUALIZED DECISION MAKING

Individualized decision making involves accounting for the risks and benefits of cancer screening among older adults, as well as perspectives and values that influence their decisions.[5] We suggest a structured framework focused on 3 key areas to develop an individualized recommendation: (1) the person's overall health and estimated life expectancy, (2) individual preferences and values, and (3) how health, life expectancy, and individual preferences impact the potential benefits and harms of screening tests. We discuss each factor in more detail as follows.

Overall Health and Life Expectancy

Clinicians should make an assessment of a person's overall health and whether an individual has a life expectancy of at least 10 years, because the harms of screening outweigh the benefits for those with less than a 10 year life expectancy.[5] There are several potential approaches to estimating health and life expectancy. First, clinicians can use their clinical judgment to determine whether an individual is in the highest quartile, middle 2 quartiles, or lowest quartile of life expectancy for their age group and match this to life table data (**Fig. 1**).[5,6] These data, for example, show that women age 80 in the top or middle 2 quartiles might benefit from cancer screening, women age 85 need to be in the top quartile of health to potentially benefit, and women age 90 are unlikely to benefit in any quartile. In addition, most men older than 85 are unlikely to benefit from cancer screening. Approaches to determining the quartile of health for each person includes conducting a clinical examination to assess gait speed,[7] self-rated health, and/or the severity of multiple chronic medical conditions.[5] For example, persons diagnosed with moderate or severe dementia on average less than a 10-year life expectancy and often cannot

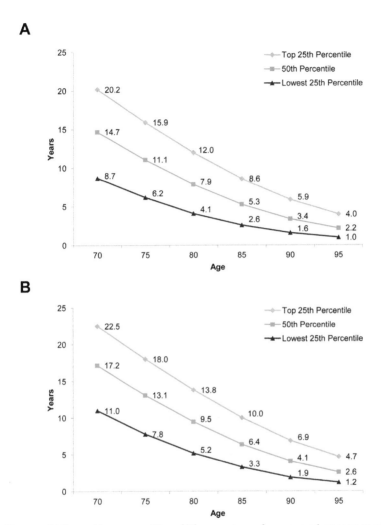

Fig. 1. Upper, middle, and lower quartiles of life expectancy for men and women at selected ages based on 2017 US life tables. (*A*) Life expectancy for men. (*B*) Life expectancy for women. (*Data is* derived from life expectancy tables in Arias E, Xu J. United States Life Tables, 2017. *National Vital Statistics Reports.* 2017;68(7).)

tolerate invasive downstream interventions. For another example, a 70-year-old with poorly controlled heart failure experiencing frequent hospitalizations is less likely to benefit from cancer screening, compared with a 77-year-old with well-controlled heart failure.

Second, clinicians can enhance their clinical judgment of estimated life expectancy by using online prognostic tools. A collection of prognostic calculators is provided online (see: eprognosis.org) that specifically estimate 10-year life expectancy (**Fig. 2A**).[8] These short online calculators include measures of age, medical conditions, functional disabilities, and health behaviors, such as smoking status, to provide percentage estimates of 10-year mortality. Having more than a 50% likelihood of 10-year mortality indicates an individual has less than a 10-year life expectancy and is unlikely to benefit from cancer screening.

A

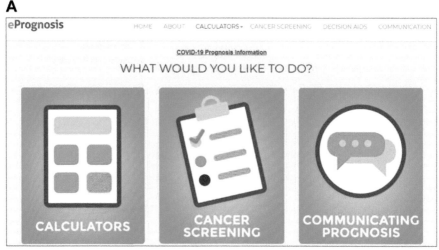

B

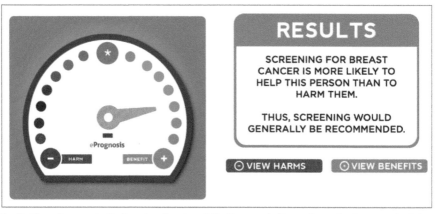

Fig. 2. The ePrognosis Online Application. (*A*) ePrognosis Home Page for Prognostic Calculators, Cancer Screening, and Communication Strategies. (*B*) Breast Cancer Screening Prognostic Calculator and Decision Support Tool. Source: www.eprognosis.org (accessed July 23, 2020). After arriving to the Web site main page (*A*), users can choose the "Cancer Screening" option, which will prompt users to select the cancer screening test they would like decision support for. Options include breast cancer screening, colorectal cancer screening, or both. After selecting a cancer screening test, users can complete an online prognostic calculator and results of this prognostic calculator are integrated into a decision support tool with multiple visual representations of data to facilitate shared decision making. An example of part of the breast cancer screening decision aid is shown in (*B*).

Individual Preferences and Values

It is important to understand a person's preferences for cancer screening and values that guide their decision making. Older adults should be asked, for example, about if they have undergone screening in the past and their experience with it. In general, clinicians can solicit perspectives on whether individuals prefer to have more medical information and testing done compared with a general preference to avoid medical testing. Individuals who feel they have other pressing health priorities might reasonably feel a need to control these conditions before pursuing cancer screening.[9] In addition, preferences include the willingness to undergo downstream invasive diagnostic procedures with a realistic understanding of potential risks and benefits. The risks of prostate biopsies, lung biopsies, or colonoscopies, for example, may not be considered tolerable to some individuals. Other individuals may have experienced false positive tests requiring biopsies in the past, and be less willing to undergo such procedures again.[10] In addition, it can be helpful to have a general sense of willingness to undergo more invasive or major treatments, such as surgery or chemotherapy. Older adults who would not want or tolerate further workup or treatment after a positive screening test should not be screened.

Risks and Benefits of Individual Cancer Screening Tests

Individualized decisions should take into account the risks and benefits of individual cancer screening tests in the context of a person's health, life expectancy and preferences. We present a brief summary of evidence related to common cancer screening tests in older adults in which individualized decisions based on life expectancy are recommended (eg, breast, prostate, colorectal, and lung cancer screening) as well as in national guidelines. We discuss how to incorporate potential risks, benefits, and guidelines of each cancer screening test into individualized decision making. Risks and benefits are further summarized in **Table 1**.

BREAST CANCER SCREENING
Potential Benefits

Trial-based evidence of benefit in older women is uncertain because RCTs of mammography for breast cancer screening included few women older than 70. Only 1 of 8 RCTs examining mammography included a small number of women 70 to 74 years old and found no reduction in breast cancer–specific mortality in this age group. No trials have included women older than 75.[11] Observational studies have shown potential benefit of screening mammography in older women, including the detection of earlier-stage breast cancer and reduced breast cancer–specific mortality, particularly for women in better health (Charlson comorbidity scores <2 or living for a median of 10 years).[12–15] However, these results should be interpreted with caution, as they may reflect effects of length-time, lead-time, or selection bias rather than a benefit of cancer screening. Simulation models have been used to generate potential benefits of mammography among older women. These estimate 1 to 2 fewer breast cancer deaths per 1000 women in their 70s screened biennially for 10 years.[16,17] In addition, mammography may detect early cancers more frequently and more accurately (higher sensitivity and specificity) in older women.[18,19] Taken together, it is reasonable to extrapolate the modest benefits of mammography to older women who have at least a 10-year life expectancy.

Potential Harms

With 1 screening mammography test, false positive results occur in approximately 7% of women age 70 to 79, and 6.5% of women age 80 to 89, which often causes anxiety or downstream testing.[20] Biopsies are recommended in 1.8% of women age 70 to 79, and 1.6% of women age 80 to 89.[20] Breast biopsies more frequently detect cancer in older adults, but may be distressing or uncomfortable, particularly in women with dementia who may not understand what is being done to them. In model-based simulation studies of overdiagnosis, rates of overdiagnosis increase as routine cancer screening continues into older ages and for women with more comorbid medical

Table 1
Benefits and harms of cancer screening among older adults

Screening	Harms	Benefits
Breast cancer screening (Mammography)	Overdiagnosis: Model-based simulations of overdiagnosis suggest rates increase with age, with rates ranging 12%–29% for women 74 y old, 17%–41% for women 80 y old, and 32%–48% for women 90 y old.[21,22] The harms of overdiagnosis increase with age due to cancer-related treatment toxicity.[23] False positive recall following mammography: Cumulative probability of 7% in adults age 70–79 and 6.5% in women age 80–89.[20] False positives are less common in older women. Biopsies: Biopsy rate of 1.8% in women age 70–79 and 1.6% in women age 80–89.[20] Other: Anxiety, distress from false positives, financial impact of screening	Breast cancer–specific mortality reduction: No RCTs showing mortality reduction in women >70. Observational studies suggest benefit for women in good health, although results may reflect lead-time, length-time, or selection bias.[12–15] Mammography is more accurate in detecting cancer in older adults.[18,19] Simulation models indicate 1–2 fewer breast cancer deaths per 1000 women in their 70s screened biennially for 10 y.[16,17] Women should have >10-y life expectancy to extrapolate the benefits of screening seen at younger ages, which may outweigh harms of screening.
CRC screening	Overdiagnosis: Low risk, ranging 0.1%–6% of screen-detected cases.[2,4,40] False positives requiring colonoscopies: Up to 23% over 10 y of annual FOBT testing.[36] Sigmoidoscopy procedural complications: inadequate depth, perforation in 0.1 per 1000 sigmoidoscopies.[37] Colonoscopy procedural complications: Gastrointestinal adverse events (26 in 1000), perforation (1 in 1000), post-polypectomy bleeding (3.6 in 1000), severe cardiac or pulmonary events (12.1 in 1000) and death (1 in 1000).[38] Colonoscopy prep: dizziness, abdominal pain, fecal incontinence, and nausea, and individuals can experience confusion and falls with sedation post-procedure.[39]	CRC-specific mortality reduction: 11%–53% CRC-specific mortality reduction with annual FOBTs[28–32]; 35% mortality reduction from sigmoidoscopies every 3–5 y.[33] No RCTs for colonoscopy, but observational studies suggest 50% reduction in incident CRCs and 50%–63% reduced CRC mortality in adults >75 y old.[34] Older adults with >10-y life expectancy are more likely to experience benefits > harms. CRC prevention: removal of colonic adenomas can reduce CRC incidence. Lag-time to benefit of removal of adenomas of 10 y.[35]

(continued on next page)

Table 1 (continued)		
Screening	Harms	Benefits
Prostate cancer screening (prostate-specific antigen [PSA] tests)	*Overdiagnosis*: Approximately 40%–60% of screen-detected cancers based on RCT data; 24 cases of overdiagnosis for 1 case of avoided prostate cancer death for age 50–69. Overdiagnosis rate increases with older age, as does cancer-treatment adverse effects including bowel dysfunction, urinary incontinence, erectile dysfunction, and premature death.[76] *False positives requiring biopsy*: 30%–40% of PSA tests.[71] *Biopsy-related complications*: anxiety, moderate to severe pain (7%) during and immediately after the procedure, moderate to severe hematuria (6%), infection requiring hospitalization (0.4%–1.3%), and hospitalizations (7%).[72–74] *Other*: Anxiety, distress from false positives	*Prostate cancer–specific mortality reduction*: RCTs of PSA screening have provided limited evidence of benefit in men >70 y old, and have not included men >75 y old. Men should have a life expectancy of at least 10–15 y to potentially experience benefits > harms from screening.
Lung cancer screening (low-dose tomography [LDCT])	*Overdiagnosis*: Can occur in 3%–9% of screen-detected cancers.[47–49] Overdiagnosis rates increase with older age and limited life expectancy. *False positives*: 39% of people in the LDCT group had at least 1 positive test result and 96% of positive results were false positives.[49] *Biopsy-related complications*: 8%–20% rate of complications after invasive diagnostic procedures.[50–52] *Other*: Burden of nodule tracking, radiation, anxiety.	*Lung cancer–specific mortality reduction*: Two RCTs of LDCTs indicate a 20%–24% lung cancer–specific mortality reduction among adults age 55–80 with >30 pack year smoking history and either currently smoke or quit within the past 15 y.[47–49] Older adults should have a 10-y life expectancy to potentially experience benefits > harms of screening.

Definitions: Overdiagnosis: detection of a cancer that would never progress to cause symptoms in a person's lifetime, which can lead to overtreatment (surgery, radiation, chemotherapy) that provides no benefits and only adverse effects.

Abbreviations: CRC, colorectal cancer; FOBT, fecal occult blood test; RCT, randomized controlled trial.

Data from Refs.[2,4,12–23,28–40,47–52,71–74,76]

conditions.[21,22] One simulation study estimated rates of overdiagnosis ranging 12% to 29% for women who stop biennial screening at 74 years old, 17% to 41% for women who stop at 80 years old, and 32% to 48% for women who stop screening at 90 years old.[22] The harms of overdiagnosis are especially relevant to older women given the increased risks of cancer-related treatment toxicity with age.[23]

Guidelines

The American Cancer Society (ACS) recommends women ≥55 have biennial screening if they have a life expectancy ≥10 years, and the ACS does not have an age cutoff to stop screening.[1] The US Preventive Services Task Force (USPSTF) recommends biennial mammograms for women 55 to 74 years, and that current evidence is insufficient about screening women ≥75 years old.[24]

Individualized Decisions

Among older women with less than a 10-year life expectancy, we recommend discussions about stopping mammography and prioritizing preventive care toward treating known health conditions or health behaviors. When older women have at least a 10-year life expectancy, we suggest discussing risks and benefits of mammography and reaching a shared decision. The harm of overdiagnosis in older women may be of most concern,[25] and so we suggest explanations of risks using concrete numbers and visual presentations of data (**Fig. 2B**).[8] The ACS recommends decision aids be used to assist in shared decision making, and a peer-reviewed decision aid with visual representations of data specific to women age 75 to 84 and ≥85 years old is available and was recently tested in an RCT.[26,27]

COLORECTAL CANCER SCREENING
Potential Benefits

Several trials have demonstrated colorectal cancer (CRC)-specific mortality benefits in older adults. Among trials of guaiac-based fecal occult blood tests (FOBTs), hereafter referred to as FOBT and distinct from fecal immunochemical tests (FIT), 4 RCTs included a combined 50,144 participating adults age 70 to 80 years old.[2] Three European trials found reductions in CRC-specific mortality of 11% to 16%,[28–30] and a large US trial found reductions of 22% to 32% overall, with a 53% reduction among adults >70 years old.[31,32] For sigmoidoscopies, the Prostate, Lung, Colorectal, and Ovarian (PLCO) cancer screening trial included 20,726 adults older than 70 years, and found a 35% reduced CRC mortality for adults age 65 to 74 when screened every 3 to 5 years.[33] For colonoscopies, considered the definitive test for detection of CRC and precancerous lesions, there are no published RCTs. However, one large prospective cohort study found adults older than 75 had a 50% reduction in incident CRC diagnoses in both the proximal and distal colon if >5 years since the last endoscopy and 63% reduction if <5 years from last endoscopy.[34] In addition, colonoscopies prevent CRC in addition to early detection of CRC, and the CRC-specific mortality lag-time to benefit of both prevention and early detection is approximately 10 years.[35]

Potential Harms

False positives can occur with FOBT or FIT screening tests; Hubbard and colleagues[36] estimated up to 23% of individuals receiving annual FOBT screenings over a 10-year period had at least 1 false positive. In cases of sigmoidoscopy, perforation (0.1 per 1000 sigmoidoscopies) is a rare complication and there can be challenges achieving adequate depth in older adults.[37] Colonoscopies have higher rates of adverse events in adults 65 or older, and include gastrointestinal adverse events (26 in 1000), perforation (1 in 1000), post-polypectomy bleeding (3.6 in 1000), severe cardiac or pulmonary events (12.1 in 1000), and death (1 in 1000).[38] Challenges with bowel prep in older adults are common and include dizziness, abdominal pain, fecal incontinence, and nausea, and individuals can experience confusion and falls with sedation post-procedure.[39] There are limited data on overdiagnosis in CRC screening, especially because CRC screening contributes to prevention of CRC. The possibility of overdiagnosis appears to be lower compared with other cancer screening tests. Autopsy studies show a rate of 2% to 3% of individuals have undiagnosed CRC unrelated to cause of death,[2] RCT data on FOBTs suggests a rate of approximately 6% in those 40 to 60 years old,[4] and a population-based study in Germany found a rate of approximately 1% in older adults.[40]

National Guidelines

Several tests are recommended for CRC screening, including high-sensitivity FOBT, FIT, multitarget stool DNA test, sigmoidoscopy, computed tomography colonography, and colonoscopy. The USPSTF recommends routine screening for adults age 55 to 75 years old, and to consider screening as an individualized decision for adults age 76 to 85 years old.[41] The ACS recommends routine screening starting at age 45, that screening continue until age 75 for individuals with more than 10 year life expectancy, that clinicians individualize decisions for adults age 76 to 85, and discourage screening for individuals older than 85 years.[42]

Individualized Decisions

Among individuals with less than a 10-year life expectancy, CRC screening should be discouraged, as the procedural risks of colonoscopy, either as a screening test, or as a diagnostic test for positive noncolonoscopy CRC screening tests, likely outweigh the benefits. We discuss communication strategies because many older adults remain enthusiastic about continuing screening even when the tests are low-value and unlikely to help them live longer.[43] CRC screening has the greatest potential for benefit among older adults if they never were screened before, they are healthy enough to undergo treatment of colorectal cancer, and/or they have at least a 10-year life expectancy. In these individuals, before an FOBT or FIT, it is important to discuss the risk of a false positive and whether individuals would be willing to undergo a colonoscopy in the event of a positive result. For colonoscopies, individuals should receive information about the procedural risks as well as the burdens of bowel prep, sedation, and need for arranging transportation in the context of an older adult's health. Decision aids are effective at improving knowledge and reducing decisional conflict,[44] and decision aids are available that are tailored to CRC screening in older adults (see **Fig. 2**B).[45]

LUNG CANCER SCREENING
Potential Benefits

Several trials have evaluated the benefits of lung cancer screening using chest radiographs or low-dose computed tomography (LDCT) among adults age 55 to 74 years. For chest radiographs, the PLCO trial found no lung cancer mortality benefit among 154,942 adults age 55 to 74 years with no eligibility requirement regarding smoking.[46] In contrast, the National Lung Cancer Screening Trial (NLST) in the United States examined the efficacy of LDCT in 53,454 participants age 55 to 74 years with a history of at least 30 pack years of smoking who were current smokers or had quit in the past 15 years. This trial found a 20% relative reduction in lung cancer mortality compared with chest radiographs alone after 6.5 years of follow-up. Extended follow-up found an overall Number Needed to Screen (NNS) of 303 to prevent 1 death from lung cancer after a lag-time of 11 years.[47] In addition, the Dutch-Belgian Lung Cancer Screening (NELSON) Trial of LDCT was conducted on 15,792 current or former smokers (quit <10 years ago) age 50 to 74 years old who had smoked at least 15 cigarettes per day for 25 years or 10 cigarettes per day for 30 years. This trial found a 24% reduction in lung-cancer–specific mortality at 10-year follow-up.[48]

Potential Harms

False positive results are common with LDCT screening; in the NLST, 39% of people in the LDCT group had at least 1 positive test result and 96% of positive results were false positives.[49] After positive tests, most individuals had follow-up imaging, 4.2% had surgical procedures, 2.2% had biopsies, and there was an 8.5% to 9.8% complication rate after invasive diagnostic procedures.[50,51] Complication rates after invasive procedures may be higher among the general population of older adults compared with the specialty centers in the NLST. One retrospective study of 344,510 individuals aged 55 to 77 years undergoing diagnostic pulmonary procedures showed complication rates of 22% (more than twice that of NLST).[52] Moreover, false positive results and complications from diagnostic interventions are higher among older adults and among those in worse health compared with those who are younger or healthier.[53–55] The reported rates of overdiagnosis ranged from 3% in the NLST trial with extended follow-up to 8.9% in the NELSON trial, although this is an area of active study.[47,48,56] Additional harms include radiation exposure, financial strain, and anxiety from false positive results.[51]

National Guidelines

The USPSTF and ACS recommend annual LDCT for lung cancer screening in adults 55 to 74 years old (or up to 80 in USPSTF guidelines) who have a 30 pack year history and currently smoke or quit within the past 15 years.[57,58] Guidelines suggest avoiding screening in older adults with a short life expectancy (<10 years) or comorbidities that would make curative surgery or cancer-directed therapies not a reasonable option.

Individualized Decisions

LDCT may be of most benefit when an older adult is at high risk of lung cancer (calculators available),[59–61] has a smoking history comparable to the NLST or NELSON trials, and has a low risk of a competing cause of death.[62] Older adults should be counseled about the possibility of frequent follow-up nodule tracking, false positive results, including lesions detected by LDCT in the thyroid and other organs, and downstream diagnostic or therapeutic medical interventions. Medicare currently requires shared decision making between individuals and their clinicians, although in practice such conversations seem to rarely occur.[63,64] The lack of shared decision making may be expected, as lung cancer screening is relatively new and clinicians may be less comfortable discussing risks and benefits. This highlights the need for more informational content or decision aids that balance the risks and benefits of lung cancer screening. A decision support pamphlet developed by the Department of Veterans Affairs is available to help educate adults about the risks and benefits of LDCT screening.[65]

PROSTATE CANCER SCREENING
Potential Benefits

RCTs of prostate-specific antigen (PSA) screening have provided limited evidence of benefit in men ≥70 years old. The US PLCO trial examined annual PSA screening over 6 years in 76,685 men aged 55 to 74 years (approximately 10,000 men older than 70),[66] and found no prostate cancer mortality reduction even at 15 years of follow-up, although there were high rates of contamination in the control arm.[67] The European

Randomized Study of Screening for Prostate Cancer (ERSPC) trial randomized men 50 to 74 years to PSA screening every 2 to 4 years and the control group received no PSA screening.[68] Results indicated an overall 20% reduction in prostate cancer–specific mortality after a lag-time of 13 years[69]; however, benefits of screening were found only among men 55 to 69 years at randomization. In addition, a recent UK trial of a single PSA screening test was conducted in 419,582 men 55 to 69 years old and found no prostate cancer–specific mortality benefit after 10 years of follow-up.[70]

Potential Harms

False positive results are common after PSA tests (30%–40% of tests) and can lead to both anxiety and unneeded prostate biopsies.[71] Prostate biopsies are associated with anxiety, moderate to severe pain (7%) during and immediately after the procedure, moderate to severe hematuria (6%), infections requiring hospitalization (0.4%–1.3%), and hospitalizations (7%).[72–74] In addition, overdiagnosis represents a significant harm because prostate cancers detected through PSA screening are typically slow growing and may remain asymptomatic during an individual's lifetime; in the ERSPC and PLCO trials, it is estimated that 40% to 60% of screen-detected cancers were cases of overdiagnosis.[75,76] Using the ERSPC data, there were approximately 24 cases of overdiagnosis for every 1 prostate cancer–related death prevented after 14 years of follow-up. Overdiagnosis of prostate cancer is associated with anxiety during watchful waiting for low-risk cancers and adverse effects from cancer-directed treatments (including prostatectomy, androgen deprivation therapy, and radiation), which include bowel dysfunction, urinary incontinence, erectile dysfunction, premature death, and others.[77]

National Guidelines

The most recent USPSTF guidelines encourage men 55 to 69 years to make an individualized decision about PSA screening after discussion with a clinician, and men older than 70 not to be screened.[78] The ACS recommends men older than 50 with at least a 10-year life expectancy have an opportunity to make an informed decision about whether to be screened after receiving information about the uncertainties, risks, and potential benefits of PSA screening.[1]

Individualized Decisions

PSA screening in men older than 70 should be rare and considered only in men with at least a 10-year to 15-year life expectancy after a shared decision. Short-term harms from prostate biopsies should be discussed, as should the substantial harm of overdiagnosis in older men using easy to understand language and visual data. Decision aids are available, and a recent systematic review of 19 decision aids found reductions in decisional conflict to screen. However, there was little evidence that decision aids facilitate shared decision making or impact screening choice.[79]

COMMUNICATING CANCER SCREENING RECOMMENDATIONS

Individualized decision making has been a recommended strategy for improving cancer screening decisions for nearly 2 decades.[5] Yet, overscreening remains common among older adults with limited life expectancy.[39,80] Conversely, screening may not be offered to older adults with inadequate prior screening (as in CRC or cervical cancer screening) or with greater than 10-year life expectancies despite potential benefit. One possible contributor to overscreening is that individuals tend to overestimate the benefits of screening and underestimate the potential harms.[81,82] This may contribute to misplaced enthusiasm for screening or requests of health providers for screening tests when they may no longer be in the patient's best interest.[80] In response, health providers might feel uncomfortable managing these expectations or having difficult conversations about life expectancy, and even order investigations they know to be unnecessary.[83] Clinicians similarly may overestimate benefits of tests,[84] or may have difficulty translating statistical or highly numerical concepts in ways that are understandable to individuals. Finally, there are limitations in time for clinicians to incorporate estimates of life expectancy into recommendations or to have careful shared decisions with older adults. Consequently, it is essential to have insight into strategies that can enhance effective communication of cancer screening recommendations.

A recent systematic review discussed several strategies to improve discussions of risks and benefits of medical tests.[85] First, using visual displays of data can improve accurate recall of conversations and comprehension among adults. Visual displays of cancer screening risk are available online (see: eprognosis.org, see **Fig. 2**) and are in several decision aids specific to older adults.[8,26] Second, it can be helpful to provide context for cancer screening outcomes in relation to competing medical priorities or risks. For example, in an individual with poorly controlled heart disease, a discussion might contextualize that interventions to control heart disease will help the individual live longer and better than cancer screening tests. Third, we suggest avoiding positive framing, or framing testing results as gains rather than losses, as it is associated with increased acceptance of harmful interventions. Positive framing can be reduced by asking questions about individual values and preferences before discussing the risks and benefits of medical tests so as to frame testing outcomes in the context of what is important to that person.

When clinicians recommend screening, this recommendation should include a clear plan for reevaluating the need to continue screening at specified time points and an explanation of what might make cancer screening less of a priority in the future. Providing anticipatory guidance might lead to more comfort with eventual stopping of cancer screening when harms outweigh the benefits.

If clinicians feel that stopping cancer screening is most appropriate for an individual, there are several phrases that can be used to improve acceptability of the recommendation and comprehension of the reasoning. For example, a survey of older adults found that phrases such as "your other health issues should take priority," "this [screening test] is not recommended for you by medical guidelines," or "you are at high risk for harms from [this screening test]," are preferred to phrases such as "you may not live long enough to benefit from [screening]."[86] Similarly, discussing that the "risks outweigh the benefits" when considering their overall health status may be more acceptable than using the term "life expectancy." Of note, although some clinicians or older adults might find it acceptable to not offer cancer screening tests when the harms clearly outweigh potential benefits,[87] we suggest open and shared decisions.

SUMMARY

Cancer screening recommendations for older adults should be individualized to account for overall health, life expectancy, values and preferences, and how these impact the risk-benefit ratio of individual cancer screening tests. Moreover, there are strategies that clinicians should consider to best communicate these recommendations, address misperceptions, and align treatment goals between clinicians and older adults. By combining the process of individualized decision making with thoughtful communication, we may be able to shift current screening trends toward ensuring older adults who may benefit have the opportunity to be screened, and those in whom harms outweigh the benefits avoid harmful screening.

CLINICS CARE POINTS

- Cancer screening recommendations should be individualized for older adults by accounting for overall health and life expectancy, values and preferences, and how these affect specific risks and benefits of cancer screening tests.
- The benefits of cancer screening are uncertain in older adults due to lack of inclusion of adults older than 75 in most RCTs.
- Harms of cancer screening in older adults include the risk of overdiagnosis, false positive results, and procedural complications from downstream diagnostic interventions.
- Older adults with less than a 10-year life expectancy are unlikely to benefit from cancer screening and may be more likely experience harms of testing.
- Communicating screening recommendations should incorporate visual data when possible, provide context in terms of competing medical priorities, and use phrases considered more acceptable and easy to understand by older adults.

DISCLOSURE

Dr. Ashwin Kotwal's effort was supported by a GEMSSTAR Award from the National Institute on Aging (R03AG064323), the NIA Claude D. Pepper Older Americans Independence Center (P30AG044281), and the National Palliative Care Research Center Kornfield Scholar's Award. Dr. Louise Walter's effort on this project was supported by a K24 Midcareer Mentoring Award for Patient-Oriented Research in Aging (K24AG041180) from the National Institute on Aging.

REFERENCES

1. Smith RA, Andrews KS, Brooks D, et al. Cancer screening in the United States, 2019: A review of current American Cancer Society guidelines and current issues in cancer screening. CA Cancer J Clin 2019;69:184–210.
2. Walter LC, Lewis CL, Barton MB. Screening for colorectal, breast, and cervical cancer in the elderly: a review of the evidence. Am J Med 2005;118(10):1078–86.
3. Kotwal AA, Schonberg MA. Cancer screening in the elderly: a review of breast, colorectal, lung, and prostate cancer screening. Cancer J 2017;23(4):246–53.
4. Carter JL, Coletti RJ, Harris RP. Quantifying and monitoring overdiagnosis in cancer screening: a systematic review of methods. BMJ 2015;350:g7773.
5. Walter LC, Covinsky KE. Cancer screening in elderly patients: a framework for individualized decision making. JAMA 2001;285(21):2750–6.
6. Arias E, Xu J. United States life tables, 2017. Natl Vital Stat Rep 2017;68(7):1–66.
7. Kotwal AA, Mohile SG, Dale W. Remaining life expectancy measurement and PSA screening of older men. J Geriatr Oncol 2012;3(3):196–204.
8. ePrognosis: Lee Schonberg Index. Available at: http://eprognosis.ucsf.edu/leeschonberg.php. Accessed April 5, 2017.
9. Schoenborn NL, Xue Q-L, Pollack CE, et al. Demographic, health, and attitudinal factors predictive of cancer screening decisions in older adults. Prev Med Rep 2019;13:244–8.

10. Dabbous FM, Dolecek TA, Berbaum ML, et al. Impact of a false-positive screening mammogram on subsequent screening behavior and stage at breast cancer diagnosis. Cancer Epidemiol Biomarkers Prev 2017;26(3):397–403.

11. Tabár L, Vitak B, Chen H-H, et al. The Swedish Two-County Trial twenty years later: updated mortality results and new insights from long-term follow-up. Radiol Clin North Am 2000;38(4):625–51.

12. McCarthy EP, Burns RB, Freund KM, et al. Mammography use, breast cancer stage at diagnosis, and survival among older women. J Am Geriatr Soc 2000; 48(10):1226–33.

13. McPherson CP, Swenson KK, Lee MW. The effects of mammographic detection and comorbidity on the survival of older women with breast cancer. J Am Geriatr Soc 2002;50(6):1061–8.

14. Jonsson H, Törnberg S, Nyström L, et al. Service screening with mammography of women aged 70–74 years in Sweden: effects on breast cancer mortality. Cancer Detect Prev 2003;27(5):360–9.

15. Coldman A, Phillips N, Wilson C, et al. Pan-Canadian study of mammography screening and mortality from breast cancer. J Natl Cancer Inst 2014;106(11): dju261.

16. Barratt A, Howard K, Irwig L, et al. Model of outcomes of screening mammography: information to support informed choices. BMJ 2005;330(7497):936.

17. Walter LC, Schonberg MA. Screening mammography in older women: a review. JAMA 2014;311(13):1336–47.

18. Carney PA, Miglioretti DL, Yankaskas BC, et al. Individual and combined effects of age, breast density, and hormone replacement therapy use on the accuracy of screening mammography. Ann Intern Med 2003;138(3):168–75.

19. Lee CS, Sengupta D, Bhargavan-Chatfield M, et al. Association of patient age with outcomes of current-era, large-scale screening mammography: analysis of data from the National Mammography Database. JAMA Oncol 2017;3(8):1134–6.

20. Nelson HD, O'Meara ES, Kerlikowske K, et al. Factors associated with rates of false-positive and false-negative results from digital mammography screening: an analysis of registry data. Ann Intern Med 2016;164(4):226–35.

21. Mandelblatt JS, Stout NK, Schechter CB, et al. Collaborative modeling of the benefits and harms associated with different US breast cancer screening strategies. Ann Intern Med 2016;164(4):215–25.

22. Van Ravesteyn NT, Stout NK, Schechter CB, et al. Benefits and harms of mammography screening after age 74 years: model estimates of overdiagnosis. J Natl Cancer Inst 2015;107(7):djv103.

23. Hurria A, Brogan K, Panageas KS, et al. Patterns of toxicity in older patients with breast cancer receiving adjuvant chemotherapy. Breast Cancer Res Treat 2005; 92(2):151–6.

24. Siu AL. Screening for breast cancer: US Preventive Services Task Force recommendation statement. Ann Intern Med 2016;164(4):279–96.

25. Hersch J, Jansen J, Barratt A, et al. Women's views on overdiagnosis in breast cancer screening: a qualitative study. BMJ 2013;346:f158.

26. Schonberg MA, Hamel MB, Davis RB, et al. Development and evaluation of a decision aid on mammography screening for women 75 years and older. JAMA Intern Med 2014;174(3):417–24.

27. Schonberg MA, Kistler CE, Pinheiro A, et al. Effect of a mammography screening decision aid for women 75 years and older: a cluster randomized clinical trial. JAMA Intern Med 2020;180(6):831–42.

28. Scholefield J, Moss S, Mangham C, et al. Nottingham trial of faecal occult blood testing for colorectal cancer: a 20-year follow-up. Gut 2012;61:1036–40.

29. Faivre J, Dancourt V, Denis B, et al. Comparison between a guaiac and three immunochemical faecal occult blood tests in screening for colorectal cancer. Eur J Cancer 2012;48(16):2969–76.

30. Kronborg O, Jørgensen O, Fenger C, et al. Randomized study of biennial screening with a faecal occult blood test: results after nine screening rounds. Scand J Gastroenterol 2004;39(9):846–51.

31. Mandel JS, Church TR, Bond JH, et al. The effect of fecal occult-blood screening on the incidence of colorectal cancer. N Engl J Med 2000;343(22):1603–7.

32. Shaukat A, Mongin SJ, Geisser MS, et al. Long-term mortality after screening for colorectal cancer. N Engl J Med 2013;369(12):1106–14.

33. Schoen RE, Pinsky PF, Weissfeld JL, et al. Colorectal-cancer incidence and mortality with screening flexible sigmoidoscopy. N Engl J Med 2012;366(25):2345–57.

34. Nishihara R, Wu K, Lochhead P, et al. Long-term colorectal-cancer incidence and mortality after lower endoscopy. N Engl J Med 2013;369(12):1095–105.

35. Zauber AG, Winawer SJ, O'Brien MJ, et al. Colonoscopic polypectomy and long-term prevention of colorectal-cancer deaths. N Engl J Med 2012;366:687–96.

36. Hubbard RA, Johnson E, Hsia R, et al. The cumulative risk of false-positive fecal occult blood test after 10 years of colorectal cancer screening. Cancer Epidemiol Biomarkers Prev 2013;22(9):1612–9.

37. Lin JS, Piper MA, Perdue LA, et al. Screening for colorectal cancer: updated evidence report and systematic review for the US Preventive Services Task Force. JAMA 2016;315(23):2576–94.

38. Day LW, Kwon A, Inadomi JM, et al. Adverse events in older patients undergoing colonoscopy: a systematic review and meta-analysis. Gastrointest Endosc 2011;74(4):885–96.

39. Schonberg MA, Breslau ES, Hamel MB, et al. Colon cancer screening in US adults aged 65 and older according to life expectancy and age. J Am Geriatr Soc 2015;63(4):750–6.

40. Brenner H, Altenhofen L, Stock C, et al. Prevention, early detection, and overdiagnosis of colorectal cancer within 10 years of screening colonoscopy in Germany. Clin Gastroenterol Hepatol 2015;13(4):717–23.

41. Bibbins-Domingo K, Grossman DC, Curry SJ, et al. Screening for colorectal cancer: US Preventive Services Task Force recommendation statement. JAMA 2016;315(23):2564–75.

42. Wolf AM, Fontham ET, Church TR, et al. Colorectal cancer screening for average-risk adults: 2018 guideline update from the American Cancer Society. CA Cancer J Clin 2018;68(4):250–81.

43. Piper MS, Maratt JK, Zikmund-Fisher BJ, et al. Patient attitudes toward individualized recommendations to stop low-value colorectal cancer screening. JAMA Netw open 2018;1(8):e185461.

44. Volk RJ, Linder SK, Lopez-Olivo MA, et al. Patient decision aids for colorectal cancer screening: a systematic review and meta-analysis. Am J Prev Med 2016;51(5):779–91.

45. Lewis CL, Golin CE, DeLeon C, et al. A targeted decision aid for the elderly to decide whether to undergo colorectal cancer screening: development and results of an uncontrolled trial. BMC Med Inform Decis Mak 2010;10(1):1.

46. Oken MM, Hocking WG, Kvale PA, et al. Screening by chest radiograph and lung cancer mortality: the Prostate, Lung, Colorectal, and Ovarian (PLCO) randomized trial. Jama 2011;306(17):1865–73.

47. National Lung Screening Trial Research Team. Lung cancer incidence and mortality with extended follow-up in the national lung screening trial. J Thorac Oncol 2019;14(10):1732–42.

48. de Koning HJ, van der Aalst CM, de Jong PA, et al. Reduced lung-cancer mortality with volume CT screening in a randomized trial. N Engl J Med 2020; 382(6):503–13.

49. Aberle D, Adams A, Berg C, et al. Reduced lung-cancer mortality with low-dose computed tomographic screening. N Engl J Med 2011;365(5):395–409.

50. Bach PB, Mirkin JN, Oliver TK, et al. Benefits and harms of CT screening for lung cancer: a systematic review. Jama 2012;307(22):2418–29.

51. Harris RP, Sheridan SL, Lewis CL, et al. The harms of screening: a proposed taxonomy and application to lung cancer screening. JAMA Intern Med 2014;174(2): 281–6.

52. Huo J, Xu Y, Sheu T, et al. Complication rates and downstream medical costs associated with invasive diagnostic procedures for lung abnormalities in the community setting. JAMA Intern Med 2019;179(3):324–32.

53. Wiener RS, Schwartz LM, Woloshin S, et al. Population-based risk for complications after transthoracic needle lung biopsy of a pulmonary nodule: an analysis of discharge records. Ann Intern Med 2011;155(3):137–44.

54. Kozower BD, Sheng S, O'brien SM, et al. STS database risk models: predictors of mortality and major morbidity for lung cancer resection. Ann Thorac Surg 2010; 90(3):875–83.

55. Pinsky PF, Gierada DS, Hocking W, et al. National Lung Screening Trial findings by age: Medicare-eligible versus under-65 population. Ann Intern Med 2014; 161(9):627–33.

56. Heleno B, Siersma V, Brodersen J. Estimation of overdiagnosis of lung cancer in low-dose computed tomography screening: a secondary analysis of the Danish lung cancer screening trial. JAMA Intern Med 2018;178(10):1420–2.

57. Moyer VA. Screening for lung cancer: US Preventive Services Task Force recommendation statement. Ann Intern Med 2014;160(5):330–8.

58. Wender R, Fontham ET, Barrera E Jr, et al. American Cancer Society lung cancer screening guidelines. CA Cancer J Clin 2013;63(2):107–17.

59. MSKCC. Lung Cancer Screening Decision Tool. 2014. Available at: http://nomograms.mskcc.org/Lung/Screening.aspx. Accessed January 27, 2017.

60. Kovalchik SA, Tammemagi M, Berg CD, et al. Targeting of low-dose CT screening according to the risk of lung-cancer death. N Engl J Med 2013;369(3):245–54.

61. Katki HA, Kovalchik SA, Berg CD, et al. Development and validation of risk models to select ever-smokers for CT lung cancer screening. Jama 2016; 315(21):2300–11.

62. Caverly TJ, Fagerlin A, Wiener RS, et al. Comparison of observed harms and expected mortality benefit for persons in the Veterans Health Affairs Lung Cancer Screening Demonstration Project. JAMA Intern Med 2018;178(3):426–8.

63. Goodwin JS, Nishi S, Zhou J, et al. Use of the shared decision-making visit for lung cancer screening among Medicare enrollees. JAMA Intern Med 2019; 179(5):716–8.

64. Brenner AT, Malo TL, Margolis M, et al. Evaluating shared decision making for lung cancer screening. JAMA Intern Med 2018;178(10):1311–6.

65. VA. Screening for Lung Cancer. 2014. Available at: http://www.prevention.va.gov/docs/LungCancerScreeningHandout.pdf. Accessed January 26, 2017.
66. Andriole GL, Crawford ED, Grubb RL III, et al. Mortality results from a randomized prostate-cancer screening trial. N Engl J Med 2009;360(13):1310–9.
67. Pinsky PF, Prorok PC, Yu K, et al. Extended mortality results for prostate cancer screening in the PLCO trial with median follow-up of 15 years. Cancer 2017; 123(4):592–9.
68. Schröder FH, Hugosson J, Roobol MJ, et al. Screening and prostate-cancer mortality in a randomized European study. N Engl J Med 2009;2009(360):1320–8.
69. Schröder FH, Hugosson J, Roobol MJ, et al. Screening and prostate cancer mortality: results of the European Randomised Study of Screening for Prostate Cancer (ERSPC) at 13 years of follow-up. Lancet 2014;384(9959):2027–35.
70. Martin RM, Donovan JL, Turner EL, et al. Effect of a low-intensity PSA-based screening intervention on prostate cancer mortality: the CAP randomized clinical trial. Jama 2018;319(9):883–95.
71. Brawer MK. Prostate-specific antigen: current status. CA Cancer J Clin 1999; 49(5):264–81.
72. Loeb S, Carter HB, Berndt SI, et al. Complications after prostate biopsy: data from SEER-Medicare. J Urol 2011;186(5):1830–4.
73. Loeb S, Vellekoop A, Ahmed HU, et al. Systematic review of complications of prostate biopsy. Eur Urol 2013;64(6):876–92.
74. Rosario DJ, Lane JA, Metcalfe C, et al. Short term outcomes of prostate biopsy in men tested for cancer by prostate specific antigen: prospective evaluation within ProtecT study. BMJ 2012;344:d7894.
75. Welch HG, Black WC. Overdiagnosis in cancer. J Natl Cancer Inst 2010;102(9): 605–13.
76. Draisma G, Etzioni R, Tsodikov A, et al. Lead time and overdiagnosis in prostate-specific antigen screening: importance of methods and context. J Natl Cancer Inst 2009;101(6):374–83.
77. Roussel B, Ouellet GM, Mohile SG, et al. Prostate cancer in elderly men: screening, active surveillance, and definitive therapy. Clin Geriatr Med 2015;31(4):615–29.
78. Grossman DC, Curry SJ, Owens DK, et al. Screening for prostate cancer: US Preventive Services Task Force recommendation statement. Jama 2018;319(18): 1901–13.
79. Riikonen JM, Guyatt GH, Kilpeläinen TP, et al. Decision aids for prostate cancer screening choice: a systematic review and meta-analysis. JAMA Intern Med 2019;179(8):1072–82.
80. Kotwal AA, Walter LC, Lee SJ, et al. Are we choosing wisely? older adults' cancer screening intentions and recalled discussions with physicians about stopping. J Gen Intern Med 2019;34(8):1538–45.
81. Schwartz LM, Woloshin S, Fowler FJ Jr, et al. Enthusiasm for cancer screening in the United States. Jama 2004;291(1):71–8.
82. Hoffmann TC, Del Mar C. Patients' expectations of the benefits and harms of treatments, screening, and tests: a systematic review. JAMA Intern Med 2015; 175(2):274–86.
83. Campbell EG, Regan S, Gruen RL, et al. Professionalism in medicine: results of a national survey of physicians. Ann Intern Med 2007;147(11):795–802.
84. Krouss M, Croft L, Morgan DJ. Physician understanding and ability to communicate harms and benefits of common medical treatments. JAMA Intern Med 2016; 176(10):1565–7.

85. Zipkin DA, Umscheid CA, Keating NL, et al. Evidence-based risk communication: a systematic review. Ann Intern Med 2014;161(4):270–80.
86. Schoenborn NL, Janssen EM, Boyd CM, et al. Preferred clinician communication about stopping cancer screening among older us adults: results from a national survey. JAMA Oncol 2018;4(8):1126–8.
87. Schoenborn NL, Boyd CM, Lee SJ, et al. Communicating about stopping cancer screening: comparing clinicians' and older adults' perspectives. Gerontologist 2019;59(Supplement_1):S67–76.

Screening for Breast Cancer

Anand K. Narayan, MD, PhD[a],*, Christoph I. Lee, MD, MS[b],
Constance D. Lehman, MD, PhD[c],[1]

KEYWORDS

- Mammography • Screening • Health care providers • Cancer screening guidelines

KEY POINTS

- Mammography screening in average risk women reduces breast cancer mortality.
- Primary care physicians need to work closely with radiologists to tailor screening programs to maximize the benefits of screening mammography while minimizing potential harms.
- Despite differences between guidelines, all guidelines agree that average risk women between the ages of 50-74 years old should undergo routine mammographic screening
- By framing false positives as part of the screening process in which additional images are occasionally required to complete the imaging evaluation, primary care providers can help reduce anxiety from recalls.
- Overdiagnosis has been identified as one of the principle harms associated with screening mammography, however widely ranging estimates present challenges to primary care practitioners trying to counsel their patients.

INTRODUCTION

Among women, breast cancer is the most commonly diagnosed cancer and the leading cause of cancer-related death in the world.[1] In the United States, breast cancer is the second leading cause of cancer death in women.[2] Nearly 40,000 women die from breast cancer every year in the United States.

Screening mammography is the most commonly used method to detect breast cancer in asymptomatic women. In the United States, every major guideline-producing organization has recommended screening mammography in average-risk women.[3] However, existing guidelines differ regarding when to start and stop and how often women should undergo screening, reflecting varying perspectives about the overall balance of benefits and harms of mammographic screening.

[a] Radiology, Massachusetts General Hospital, 55 Fruit Street, Wang 240, Boston, MA 02114, USA; [b] Department of Radiology, Department of Health Services, Northwest Screening and Cancer Outcomes Research Enterprise, University of Washington, 1144 Eastlake Avenue East, LG-212, Seattle, WA 98109, USA; [c] Radiology, Harvard Medical School, Massachusetts General Hospital, 55 Fruit Street, Wang Building, Suite 219L, Boston, MA 02114, USA
[1] Senior author.
* Corresponding author.
E-mail address: AKNARAYAN@mgh.harvard.edu
Twitter: @AnandKNarayan (A.K.N.)

Med Clin N Am 104 (2020) 1007–1021
https://doi.org/10.1016/j.mcna.2020.08.003
medical.theclinics.com

This article reviews the evidence regarding breast cancer screening for average-risk women. The review primarily focuses on mammographic screening but also reviews clinical breast examinations, emerging screening technologies, and opportunities to build consensus. Wherever possible, the review relies on published systematic reviews, meta-analyses, and guidelines from three major societies (US Preventive Services Task Force [USPSTF], American College of Radiology [ACR], and the American Cancer Society [ACS]) to reflect a range of evidence-based perspectives regarding mammographic screening.

GUIDELINE DEVELOPMENT METHODS

The USPSTF is a volunteer panel of 16 nationally recognized experts in primary care, prevention, and evidence-based medicine. Details regarding guideline development methods are described elsewhere.[4] Briefly, the USPSTF screening recommendations are informed by the Agency for Healthcare Research and Quality's designated Evidence Based Practice Centers, which develop evidence reviews and summaries. For the most recent breast cancer screening recommendations, the USPSTF reviewed evidence summaries generated by the Pacific Northwest Evidence-based Practice Center.

The ACR guideline development process includes reviewing and analyzing the current, peer-reviewed medical literature. The ACR process uses scientific evidence review and expert consensus. Experts in diagnostic imaging, interventional radiology, and radiation oncology develop ACR guidelines with participation from additional specialty societies. The ACR literature synthesis process uses the RAND/UCLA Appropriateness Method.[5] Recommendations are classified using the Grading of Recommendations Assessment, Development, and Evaluation framework.[6]

The ACS 2015 breast cancer screening guidelines were developed following standard methodologies used in ACS guidelines based on the Institute of Medicine.[7] The ACS created an interdisciplinary guideline development group (GDG) composed of clinicians, biostatisticians, epidemiologists, patient representatives, and an economist. The GDG selected the Duke University Evidence Synthesis Group to conduct an independent systematic evidence review of the breast cancer screening literature and provide recommendations based on the Grading of Recommendations Assessment, Development, and Evaluation framework.

BENEFITS OF EARLY DETECTION THROUGH MAMMOGRAPHIC SCREENING

Mammographic screening reduces breast cancer mortality according to results using a wide variety of study designs (**Fig. 1**). By limiting confounding, randomized control trials (RCTs) represent the gold standard study design for evaluating the efficacy of health care interventions. Although the specific methods of RCTs have varied widely and RCTs have limitations for diseases with long-term outcomes, they are considered the most rigorous method for testing hypotheses.[8]

The USPSTF conducted a systematic review and meta-analysis of RCTs to provide the USPSTF with updated evidence to inform their guidelines about the benefits of screening mammography.[9] For average-risk women, the systematic review and meta-analysis evaluated the effectiveness of screening mammography in reducing breast cancer mortality, all-cause mortality, and advanced breast cancer. Additionally, the systematic review evaluated how the effectiveness of screening mammography may vary by age, risk factors, and screening intervals.

Eight mammography screening trials met inclusion criteria for study quality with differing randomization, recruitment, and screening protocols. More than 600,000

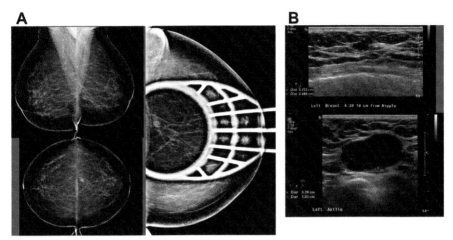

Fig. 1. (A) A 51-year-old woman presenting for screening mammogram. Patient was found to have a focal asymmetry in the left lower outer breast, which persisted on additional spot compression views. (B) Focused ultrasound of the left breast found a 0.8-cm mass at the 4:30 position, 10 cm from the nipple. Patient also noted palpable lump in the left axilla before diagnostic examination and was found to have suspicious left axillary lymph node. Both masses were biopsied revealing triple-negative breast cancer with axillary metastasis. Patient received three cycles of chemotherapy, bilateral mastectomies, left-sided axillary dissection, and radiation. Patient has demonstrated no evidence of disease after 6 years of follow-up.

women were included from the Health Insurance Plan of Greater New York trial; the Canadian National Breast Cancer Screening (CNBSS)-1 and -2 studies; the Age trial, based in the United Kingdom; and four trials based in Sweden (Stockholm trial, Malmö Mammographic Screening Trials, Gothenburg trial, and the Swedish Two-County Trial). Three trials provided longer term clinical follow-up updates (CNBSS-1 and -2, the Age trial, and the Swedish Two-County Trial). All of these trials had breast cancer mortality as their primary outcome measure. Differences between screening and control groups were evaluated following the intention-to-treat principle to reduce confounding.

The ACS review of meta-analyses found that breast cancer screening reduces breast cancer mortality after approximately 13 years of follow-up.[10] Pooled estimates for relative breast cancer mortality reductions were similar for meta-analyses using random-effects models (UK Independent Panel: relative risk [RR], 0.80; 95% confidence interval [CI], 0.73–0.89; Canadian Task Force: RR, 0.82; 95% CI, 0.74–0.94) and the fixed-effects model (Cochrane analysis: RR, 0.81; 95% CI, 0.74–0.87).

Meta-analyses of RCTs have been the primary source of evidence supporting the benefit of screening mammography in guideline development, because observational studies evaluating breast cancer screening must be interpreted with caution because of susceptibility to biases including selection bias, lead time bias, length bias, and several others. However, most RCTs were conducted decades ago and evaluated the efficacy of screen film mammography using older technology and protocols that are not used today. Furthermore, the estimate of efficacy is based on intention-to-treat analyses, which means that breast cancer deaths among women in the invited group who never attended screening are still attributed to the screening arm. With the dissemination of digital mammography and rapid advances in breast imaging technologies, and the interest in measuring the effectiveness of mammography screening among women who attend screening, the ACS concluded that large, methodologically rigorous observational studies can provide valuable information about the contemporary effectiveness of screening mammography.[10] The main observational study designs reviewed included temporal studies comparing changes in breast cancer mortality before and after the introduction of breast cancer screening, incidence-based mortality studies comparing mortality rates of women who were screened or were invited to screen with women who were not screened or were not invited to screening, and case-control studies comparing histories of women who died of breast cancer compared with women who did not die from breast cancer. Temporal studies evaluating breast cancer mortality rates before and after the introduction of mammography screening programs have reported risk reductions ranging from 28% to 36%.[11] Incidence-based mortality studies found that women invited to breast cancer screening experienced a 25% reduction in breast cancer mortality (RR, 0.75; 95% CI, 0.69–0.81) and a 38% reduction in breast cancer mortality among those who attended screening (RR, 0.62; 95% CI, 0.56–0.69). Finally, pooled estimates from case control studies found that screening was associated with a 31% reduction in breast cancer mortality (odds ratio [OR], 0.69; 95% CI, 0.57–0.83), and a 48% reduction in breast cancer mortality (OR, 0.52; 95% CI, 0.42–0.65) after adjustment for self-selection. Overall, the ACS GDG deemed the strength of evidence that being invited or exposed to screening mammography reduces breast cancer mortality to be high.

HARMS ASSOCIATED WITH MAMMOGRAPHIC SCREENING, DIAGNOSIS, AND TREATMENT

The USPSTF conducted a systematic review and meta-analysis to estimate the potential harms of mammography screening including false-positive mammography results, overdiagnosed/overtreated breast cancers, anxiety, pain during procedures, and radiation exposure.[12] Additionally, they considered the extent to which these potential harms may vary by age, risk factors, and screening intervals. Their systematic review included 59 studies addressing key outcomes including 10 systematic reviews of 134 studies and 49 additional studies. Of these harms, the USPSTF identified two major potential harms associated with screening mammography: overdiagnosis/overtreatment and false positives.

Overdiagnosis

According to the USPSTF, overdiagnosis/overtreatment is the principal harm associated with screening mammography. Overdiagnosis/overtreatment refers to the diagnosis and treatment of breast cancers that would not cause harm during a patient's lifetime because these cancers would progress too slowly, not progress at all, or resolve spontaneously. It is important to stress that there is no ability to directly observe overdiagnosis, that is, to distinguish a truly nonprogressive cancer from one that is progressive, and thus the rate of overdiagnosis can only be statistically estimated by comparing incidence rates over time in groups exposed and unexposed to mammography screening.[13] This is challenging because in a group exposed to mammography, lead time significantly increases incidence rates, and over time, as women increase in age, and sojourn times lengthen, the effect of lead time on incidence rates increases, giving the spurious impression of considerable overdiagnosis in the screened arm compared with the unscreened arm.[13]

The USPSTF review for the outcome of overdiagnosis/overtreatment identified one meta-analysis of three RCTs, a systematic review of 13 observational studies, and 18 individual observational studies published since systematic reviews were conducted.

Studies used different measures of overdiagnosis/overtreatment and differing assumptions about incidence rates.

The USPSTF systematic review of 13 observational studies found estimates of overdiagnosis/overtreatment percentages ranging between 0% and 54%. Of these studies, studies that adjusted for underlying breast cancer risk, potential confounders, and lead time estimated overdiagnosis/overtreatment percentages ranging between 1% and 10%.[13]

According to the USPSTF and the Independent UK report on Mammography Screening,[14] data from RCTs offer the least biased method for estimating overdiagnosis associated with breast cancer screening. Long-term follow-up data of three RCTs (the Malmö I trial, CNBSS-1, and CNBSS-2) found percentages of overdiagnosed/overtreated cases ranging from 11% and 22%. However, Njor and colleagues[15] identified factors in the post-trial period of each of these trials that rendered these estimates unreliable.

Regardless of the study design, the ACS GDG concluded that the quality of evidence was high that overdiagnosis/overtreatment exists as a consequence of mammographic screening. However, given the widely ranging estimates, the GDG concluded that the quality of evidence for estimating the precise proportion of overdiagnosed/overtreated cases was low. Widely ranging estimates about the magnitude and extent of overdiagnosis/overtreatment present challenges to health care providers who are attempting to provide accurate information about the potential harms of mammographic screening. However, because most women are not diagnosed with breast cancer in their lifetime, the risk of being diagnosed with a nonprogressive cancer is low. The Independent UK Panel on Breast Cancer Screening estimated that of approximately 307,000 women between the ages of 50 and 52 years old invited to begin mammographic screening every year, only 1% would be diagnosed with an overdiagnosed cancer over the next 20 years.[14]

False Positives

The USPSTF systematic review identified two observational studies that estimated the cumulative probability of false-positive results after 10 years of screening with film and digital mammography, based on data from the Breast Cancer Surveillance Consortium (BCSC),[16] a collaborative network of eight breast imaging registries across the United States. They estimated the probability of receiving at least one false-positive mammography result over the course of a 10-year period for women undergoing mammography screening every year or every 2 years either starting at age 40 or age 50.[17] Cumulative probabilities were the same for annual mammography (61%) versus biennial mammography (42%) for women starting screening at age 40 versus age 50 (**Fig. 2**). Similarly, cumulative false-positive biopsy recommendations were higher for women undergoing annual screening versus biennial screening, for women starting at age 40 (7% vs 5%) and women starting at age 50 (9% vs 6%) (**Fig. 3**).

In stratified analyses, they found that false-positive mammography results and rates of false-positive biopsies were highest among women receiving annual mammography, women between the ages of 40 and 49 years old, women with extremely dense breast tissue, and/or women using combination hormone therapy.[18]

To evaluate consequences of false-positive examinations, USPSTF's systematic review found four systematic reviews of 70 unique studies and 10 additional observational studies that described the adverse effects of mammographic screening. Many of these studies were limited by small sample sizes, narrow participant selection, generalizability, and variability in outcome measures. The review cited eight studies that found that false-positive results led only to transient anxiety in most

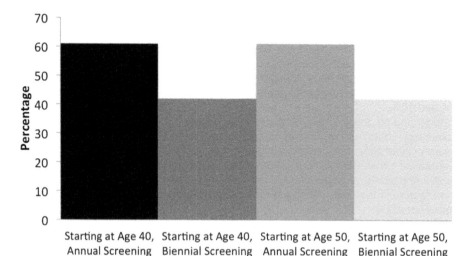

Fig. 2. Breast Cancer Surveillance Consortium estimates of 10-year cumulative probability of obtaining at least one false-positive result under different screening strategies (starting at age 40 vs starting at age 50; annual vs biennial screening).

women, whereas citing five studies that found that false-positive results led to persistent anxiety in some women, ranging between 3 months and 3 years after false-positive results. The review found two studies that concluded that women were less likely to return for screening mammography after false-positive results, two studies that found no differences in reattendance rates after false-positive results, and one study that reported an increase in attendance rates after false-positive results. Of all

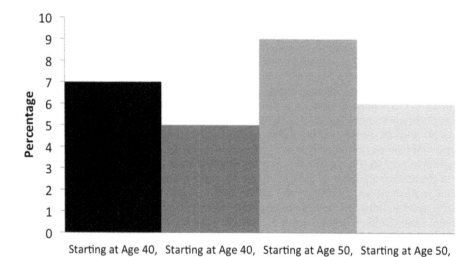

Fig. 3. Breast Cancer Surveillance Consortium estimates of 10-year cumulative probability of at least one false-positive biopsy recommendation under different screening strategies (starting at age 40 vs starting at age 50; annual vs biennial screening).

these studies, one was nested within an RCT, the Digital Mammographic Imaging Screening Trial (DMIST) comparing full field digital mammography with conventional film-screen mammography.[19] Tosteson and colleagues[19] evaluated quality of life in DMIST patients shortly after undergoing mammography screening and 1 year later using the Spielberger State-Trait Anxiety Inventory state scale and the EuroQol EQ-5D instrument. They found women with false-positive results were more likely to experience short-term anxiety but found no statistically significant differences in anxiety or overall health-related quality of life after 1 year of follow-up. Additionally, women with false-positive mammography results were more likely to state that they would undergo screening mammography in the future (OR, 2.12; 95% CI, 1.54–2.93), and most women reported that they would not be willing to travel a longer distance to reduce their chance of having a false-positive mammogram. Overall, the USPSTF concluded that although the effects of anxiety from mammographic screening may cause harms, the absolute magnitude and time course of anxiety experienced by individual women were difficult to estimate and varied widely.

Primary care doctors play a critical role ensuring that patients remain up to date with screening mammography.[20] For primary care doctors who will be counseling their patients about screening mammography, the results of these studies provide helpful guidance for patients who may be concerned about tradeoffs between potential benefits and harms associated with screening mammography. For women preparing to undergo screening mammography, women should be counseled that being recalled from screening mammography occurs commonly in the United States. Depending on the frequency of mammographic screening, approximately half of women are recalled at least once over a 10-year period. In particular, recalls are highest for women who are undergoing their first screening mammograms and women with dense breast tissue.[18] The experience of being recalled for further evaluation is stressful in the short term; however, for most women, most recalls from screening mammography turn out to be normal.[21] By framing false positives associated with screening mammography as part of a continuous portion of the screening process in which additional images are occasionally required to complete the imaging evaluation, primary care providers can help reduce anxiety associated with recalls from screening mammography. Patients should be reassured that the anxiety caused by false-positive examinations is considered short-term and not associated with long-term anxiety or health utility decrement.[19]

CURRENT GUIDELINES

With evidence from RCTs that screening mammography reduces breast cancer mortality, every major guideline-producing organization in the United States has recommended screening mammography in average-risk women.[3] However, guideline-producing organizations have offered differing recommendations about when to start and stop and how often women should undergo mammographic screening. For start age and frequency, recommendations range from annual mammographic screening starting at age 40 (ACR) to biennial mammographic screening between the ages of 50 and 74 years old (USPSTF) to annual mammographic screening starting at age 45 (ACS) (**Fig. 4**). We describe the varying perspectives regarding the overall balance of benefits and harms of breast cancer screening used to inform each screening guideline recommendation.

US Preventive Services Task Force

In 2016, the USPSTF recommended that women between the ages of 50 and 74 years old undergo mammographic screening every 2 years.[22] They concluded

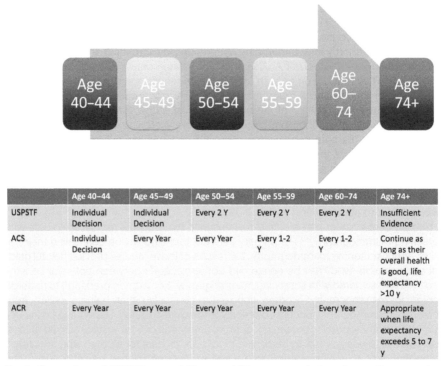

	Age 40–44	Age 45–49	Age 50–54	Age 55–59	Age 60–74	Age 74+
USPSTF	Individual Decision	Individual Decision	Every 2 Y	Every 2 Y	Every 2 Y	Insufficient Evidence
ACS	Individual Decision	Every Year	Every Year	Every 1-2 Y	Every 1-2 Y	Continue as long as their overall health is good, life expectancy >10 y
ACR	Every Year	Every Year	Every Year	Every Year	Every Year	Appropriate when life expectancy exceeds 5 to 7 y

Fig. 4. Comparison of USPSTF versus ACS versus ACR recommendations for routine screening mammography by age category.

that women between the ages of 40 and 49 years old should make individual decisions about starting breast cancer screening. For women between the ages of 40 and 49 who place higher value of the potential benefits of breast cancer screening over the potential harms, the USPSTF recommended mammographic screening every 2 years.

In determining their recommendation that average-risk women should routinely start mammographic screening at age 50, the USPSTF noted that most of the benefit of mammographic screening results from biennial screening during ages 50 to 74 years.[22] Although noting that mammographic screening in women between the ages of 40 and 49 may reduce breast cancer mortality, they noted that comparatively smaller numbers of breast cancer deaths were averted by starting screening at age 40 instead of age 50, whereas the number of false-positive results and unnecessary biopsies increased by starting screening at age 40.

The USPSTF found that current evidence is insufficient to assess the benefits and harms for women aged 75 years or older, citing a lack of RCT data in women in this age group. However, they cited CISNET modeling studies suggesting that screening women older than 74 years old may be beneficial among women with no or low comorbidity.

American College of Radiology

The ACR reviewed RCTs and meta-analyses and recommended annual mammography screening beginning at 40 years of age.[23] In their review, they cited results from RCTs finding that breast cancer screening in women starting at age 40 reduces the most deaths from breast cancer. Additionally, women in their 40s have longer life expectancies than women in their 50s to 70s, hence screening women in their 40s produces larger gains in life years compared with screening strategies in which breast cancer screening starts at age 50.[24] Finally, they noted challenges associated with personalized screening approaches based on existing risk models. To date, there are no RCT results evaluating risk-based screening strategies. Moreover, approximately 70% to 80% of breast cancers occur in women without identifiable risk factors, suggesting that personalized screening approaches may lead to a large proportion of breast cancer cases being missed.

The ACR did not set an upper age limit for eligibility for mammographic screening. Similar to the USPSTF, they noted that there are no RCT results to inform recommendations for women greater than 74 years old. However, they cited data suggesting that mammographic screening would offer comparable performance before and after women turned 74 years old. Studies evaluating the performance of mammographic screening in women greater than 74 years old found that sensitivity and specificity of screening mammography increases with increasing age. Epidemiologic life tables suggest that large percentages of women greater than age 74 have expected life spans greater than 6 years. With results from RCTs suggesting that the benefits of screening mammography may take anywhere between 5 and 7 years to develop, the ACR recommended that women continue mammographic screening as long as their life expectancy exceeds 5 to 7 years.

American Cancer Society

The ACS GDG noted that existing RCTs were not designed to specifically evaluate hypotheses about when women should start and stop screening mammography or how often they should undergo mammographic screening. To help determine when and how often women undergo mammographic screening in the absence of RCT data, the ACS commissioned the BCSC to evaluate the association between poor prognosis breast cancer outcomes and screening intervals (every year vs every other year) and menopausal status (premenopausal vs postmenopausal).[25] Analyses stratified by menopausal status found that premenopausal women who underwent mammographic screening every 2 years were more likely to have advanced stage (stage IIB or higher) breast cancers (RR, 1.28; 95% CI, 1.01–1.63), tumor sizes greater than 15 mm (RR, 1.21; 95% CI, 1.07–1.37), and any index of poor prognosis breast cancer at diagnosis (RR, 1.11; 95% CI, 1.00–1.22) compared with premenopausal women who underwent mammographic screening every year. In contrast, postmenopausal women not taking hormone-replacement therapy undergoing screening every 2 years demonstrated no statistically significant increases in advanced-stage breast cancers or any index of poor prognosis breast cancer (RR, 1.03; 95% CI, 0.95–1.12; $P = .45$) in comparison with women undergoing screening every year. Postmenopausal women not taking hormone-replacement therapy undergoing screening every 2 years instead of every year demonstrated a borderline statistically significantly increased risk of tumors greater than 15 mm (RR, 1.11; 95% CI, 1.00–1.22; $P = .045$), whereas postmenopausal women taking hormone-replacement therapy demonstrated nonstatistically significant increases in risk of tumors greater than 15 mm (RR, 1.13; 95% CI, 0.98–1.31; $P = .09$), positive lymph nodes (RR, 1.18; 95% CI, 0.98–1.42; $P = .09$), and any index of poor prognosis breast cancer (RR, 1.12; 95% CI, 1.00–1.25; $P = .05$).

To provide precise screening recommendations, the ACS GDG examined breast cancer morbidity and mortality by 5-year age categories. They noted that prior analyses obscured important differences and similarities by restricting analyses to 10-year age categories. Using several key breast cancer outcomes (5-year breast cancer

Table 1
Key breast cancer outcomes

Age Category	5-Year Breast Cancer Risk	Proportion of All Incident Breast Cancers (%)	Distribution of Breast Cancer Deaths by Age at Diagnosis (%)	Person-Years of Life Lost at 20 Years Follow-Up
40–44	0.6	6	7	12
45–49	0.9	10	10	15
50–54	1.1	12	11	15

risk, proportion of all incident breast cancers, the distribution of breast cancer deaths, and person-years of life lost) (**Table 1**), women within the age categories of 45 to 49 years old were found to experience similar degrees of morbidity and mortality from breast cancer compared with women in the 50 to 54 age category. In contrast, women between the ages of 40 and 44 demonstrated less morbidity and mortality from breast cancer compared with women in either of those categories (45–49 and 50–54). As a result, the ACS GDG provided differing breast cancer screening recommendations based on 5-year age categories.

To balance the potential benefits of annual screening in premenopausal women with higher rates of false positives associated with more frequent screening, the ACS GDG recommended that average-risk women between the ages of 45 and 54 years old should be screened annually and women between the ages of 40 and 44 years old who choose to initiate breast cancer screening should undergo annual screening mammography. Because the GDG evidence review found comparatively fewer benefits of annual screening mammography in women after menopause, the ACS recommended that starting at age 55 (the age at which most women are postmenopausal), average-risk women should transition to mammographic screening every 2 years or have the opportunity to continue screening every year.

Regarding average-risk women beyond the age of 74, the ACS GDG noted the paucity of RCT data to inform recommendations about routine screening, similar to the USPSTF and the ACR. Nevertheless, the ACS GDG noted that age is one of the most important risk factors for breast cancer and that women between the ages of 75 and 79 demonstrate the highest breast cancer incidence rates compared with women in any other age category. Additionally, 26% of breast cancer deaths are attributable to breast cancer diagnoses after the age of 74. Consequently, the ACS recommended that women continue screening mammography if their overall health is good and they have a life expectancy of 10 years or longer.

CLINICAL BREAST EXAMINATION

The USPSTF determined that the current evidence is insufficient to evaluate the benefits and harms of the clinical breast examination.[26] Although acknowledging that clinical breast examinations are inexpensive, they noted that few studies have compared clinical breast examinations with no screening and no studies have compared clinical breast examination in combination with mammographic screening with mammographic screening alone. In their review, they found that the specificity of clinical breast examination ranged from 88% to 99% in comparison with mammography screening with specificities ranging between 94% and 97%. As a result, they cited theoretic harms associated with false-positive results from clinical breast examinations with lower specificities. However, they emphasized the lack of data available to fully evaluate the potential harms associated with clinical breast examinations.

Similar to the USPSTF, the ACS GDG acknowledged the limitations of the literature on this topic. They performed a supplemental search to identify performance characteristics associated with clinical breast examinations. They found that the addition of clinical breast examination detected only a small number of additional breast cancers (2%–6%) compared with mammographic screening alone. Additionally, they concluded that there was moderate quality evidence that adding clinical breast examinations to mammography screening increases false-positive rates. Because clinical breast examinations consume valuable time during typical clinical visits without evidence of clear benefits, the ACS GDG recommended against routine clinical examinations for breast cancer screening for average-risk women at any age group. However, the ACS stated that women should be aware of how their breasts normally look and feel. Women should notify their health care providers if they notice any changes, particularly in between regular mammograms.

Instead of performing routine clinical breast examinations, the ACS GDG recommended that clinicians use this time to ascertain family history, counsel women about the importance of being aware of changes within their own breasts, and counsel women about the potential benefits and harms of screening mammography. Accurate family histories are integral components for evaluating breast cancer risk.[27] ACS guidelines about breast cancer screening pertain to average-risk women, hence using these guidelines requires health care providers to assess whether or not their patients are low, average, or high risk. The American Society of Clinical Oncology provides guidance for practitioners to collect key components required to accurate estimate patient's breast cancer risk because of family history.[28] Minimum family history elements include: first- and second-degree maternal and paternal family history, type of primary cancer, age at diagnosis, and ethnicity. In addition to collecting these data elements, they noted that family histories should be taken at the time of diagnosis and updated periodically, because family history may evolve or become more apparent over time.

OPPORTUNITIES TO BUILD CONSENSUS

Ideally, RCTs would help investigators answer specific research questions that inform current controversies about screening mammography. The ongoing Tomosynthesis Mammographic Imaging Screening Trial (TMIST) aims to enroll 165,000 women in a trial comparing tomosynthesis with conventional two-dimensional (2D) mammography.[29] By collecting blood and buccal samples, the trials aim to help individually tailor decisions about breast cancer screening based on breast density, risk factors, and genomics. Because differences in breast cancer mortality may take nearly a decade to develop, the primary outcome for TMIST is the development of advanced breast cancer as a surrogate for breast cancer mortality. Given the costs, time, and resources required, new RCTs with breast cancer mortality as a primary end point are unlikely to resolve these research questions. Although observational studies will continue to provide valuable contributions to debates about screening mammography, health care providers will need to use existing data to help patients make informed decisions about when and how often they should undergo mammographic screening.

Using their professional knowledge of the field, the principal investigators of BCSC sites recruited 10 expert radiologists from academic and community based practices.[30] They used modified Angoff methods to determine performance benchmarks for acceptable recall rates (5%–12%) and specificities (88%–95%). BCSC data revealed wide performance variation with only 59% of radiologists having acceptable recall rates and only 63% of radiologists having acceptable specificities.[30] The ACS emphasized the need for clinicians and researchers to develop strategies to minimize the harms of false-positive examinations from screening mammography, noting the high frequency of false-positive examination results in the United States.

Technological advances have improved the performance of screening mammography over the last few decades. Prior clinical trials used film-screen techniques to evaluate the benefits of screening mammography. Since then, film-screen mammography has been replaced by digital mammography in the United States.[31] Results from DMIST found no differences in sensitivity between digital and film-screen mammography.[32] In particular, the trial found that digital mammography performed better in premenopausal women, perimenopausal women, and women with dense breasts.

Since then, the development of digital breast tomosynthesis (DBT) offers the possibility of reducing false positives while also reducing false negatives. The USPSTF described DBT as a "promising new technology," but found insufficient evidence to recommend DBT routinely. Similarly, ACS GDG stated that they had insufficient evidence at the time of their protocol review to recommend DBT for average-risk women. Alternatively, the ACR determined DBT to be "usually appropriate" for average-risk women, finding that DBT addresses some of the limitations of standard 2D mammography screening. Since the publication of these guidelines, a meta-analysis of 17 studies including 1,009,790 participants was published in 2018 comparing DBT with standard 2D examinations in the United States and Europe.[33] In the United States, implementation of DBT reduced recall rates from 11.3% to 8.0% (29% recall rate reduction) while increasing the overall cancer detection rate from 4.5 to 5.7 cancers per 1000 (27% increase).[33] Implementing strategies, such as DBT, that reduce recall rates to the lower end of BCSC performance benchmarks can substantially reduce potential harms from screening mammography.[34]

Women with dense breast tissue represent particular challenges for breast imaging practices. Breast density represents an independent risk factor for breast cancer and increased breast parenchymal density masks underlying cancers, reducing mammographic sensitivity.[35] In the meta-analysis of DBT versus 2D mammography, Marinovich and colleagues[33] found nonstatistically significant trends suggestive of improved performance of DBT in women with dense breast tissue; however, they noted that the meta-analysis was likely underpowered to adequately evaluate this association. Supplemental screening with breast MRI may offer benefits for select groups of women with dense breast tissue. A multicenter RCT in the Netherlands found that supplemental screening with breast MRI in women with extremely dense breast tissue was associated with the diagnosis of fewer interval cancers compared with mammography alone.[36] Comparing DBT with abbreviated breast MRI in women with dense breast tissue, abbreviated breast MRI was associated with a significantly higher rate of invasive breast cancer detection.[37] These results suggest that breast MRI may be able to overcome some of the limitations of 2D or DBT mammographic screening in select groups of high-risk women and women with dense breast tissue.

In addition to technological advances and measuring interpretative performance, radiology practices can implement strategies to reduce harms associated with false positives from mammographic screening. Batch reading of screening mammograms is associated with reduced recall rates with comparable cancer detection rates.[38] Radiology practices can consider offering same-day screening reads for patients who are at higher risk for false-positive examinations (eg, patients undergoing baseline examinations) or for patients or providers who are concerned about the effects of false-positive examinations.[39] For the fraction of patients who end up with biopsy recommendations, offering same-day biopsies can reduce the length of time patients spend worrying about biopsy results.[40] Finally, Lehman and colleagues[41] used artificial intelligence algorithms to help reduce variability in breast density assessment. Radiology practices may be able to use artificial intelligence algorithms to improve performance and reduce variation in mammography performance. By adopting several of these interventions, radiology practices can maximize the benefits of screening mammography while reducing potential harms.

SUMMARY

Breast cancer is the second leading cause of cancer death among women in the United States and mammography screening in average-risk women is known to reduce breast cancer mortality. Even though guidelines differ regarding when to start and stop and how often women should be screened with mammography, all guideline-producing organizations agree that women age 50 to 74 of average risk should undergo routine screening. Both the ACS and ACR also recommend annual screening among premenopausal women of average risk. Health care providers and policy makers should improve engagement with millions of women for whom these different organizations have broad consensus to increase routine screening rates while working together to develop concrete strategies to maximize the benefits of mammographic screening and minimize the harms.

DISCLOSURE

Dr. Narayan AK has Nothing to Disclose. Dr. Lee CI receives textbook royalties from McGraw Hill, Inc., Wolters Kluwer, and Oxford University Press; personal fees for journal editorial board work from the American College of Radiology; and consulting fees from GRAIL, Inc. for service on a data safety monitoring board; all outside the submitted work. He is also supported in part by the National Cancer Institute (2P01 CA154292). Dr. Lehman CD receives support from the Breast Cancer Research Foundation for her efforts in AI applied to the early detection of breast cancer.

REFERENCES

1. The Lancet. GLOBOCAN 2018: counting the toll of cancer. Lancet 2018; 392(10152):985.

2. Howlader N, Noone AM, Krapcho M, et al, editors. SEER cancer statistics review, 1975-2016. Bethesda (MD): National Cancer Institute; 2019. based on November 2018 SEER data submission, posted to the SEER web site. Available at: https:// seer.cancer.gov/csr/1975_2016/.

3. Narayan AK, Lehman CD. Mammography screening guideline controversies: opportunities to improve patient engagement in screening. J Am Coll Radiol 2020; 17(5):633–6.

4. Harris RP, Helfand M, Woolf SH, et al, Methods Work Group, Third US Preventive Services Task Force. Current methods of the US Preventive Services Task Force: a review of the process. Am J Prev Med 2001;20(3 Suppl):21–35.

5. Fitch K, Bernstein SJ, Aguilar MD, et al. The RAND/UCLA appropriateness method user's manual. Santa Monica (CA): RAND Corporation; 2001. Also available in print form. Available at: https://www.rand.org/pubs/monograph_reports/ MR1269.html.

6. Guyatt GH, Oxman AD, Vist GE, et al, GRADE Working Group. GRADE: an emerging consensus on rating quality of evidence and strength of recommendations. BMJ 2008;336(7650):924–6.

7. Brawley O, Byers T, Chen A, et al. New American Cancer Society process for creating trustworthy cancer screening guidelines. JAMA 2011;306(22):2495–9.
8. Akobeng AK. Understanding randomised controlled trials. Arch Dis Child 2005; 90(8):840–4.
9. Nelson HD, Fu R, Cantor A, et al. Effectiveness of breast cancer screening: systematic review and meta-analysis to update the 2009 U.S. Preventive Services Task Force Recommendation. Ann Intern Med 2016;164(4):244–55.
10. Oeffinger KC, Fontham ET, Etzioni R, et al, American Cancer Society. Breast cancer screening for women at average risk: 2015 guideline update from the American Cancer Society. JAMA 2015;314(15):1599–614.
11. Broeders M, Moss S, Nyström L, et al. The impact of mammographic screening on breast cancer mortality in Europe: a review of observational studies. J Med Screen 2012;19(Suppl 1):14–25.
12. Nelson HD, Pappas M, Cantor A, et al. Harms of breast cancer screening: systematic review to update the 2009 U.S. Preventive Services Task Force Recommendation. Ann Intern Med 2016;164(4):256–67.
13. Puliti D, Duffy SW, Miccinesi G, et al. Overdiagnosis in mammographic screening for breast cancer in Europe: a literature review. J Med Screen 2012;19(Suppl 1): 42–56.
14. Marmot MG, Altman DG, Cameron DA, et al. The benefits and harms of breast cancer screening: an independent review. Br J Cancer 2013;108:2205–40.
15. Njor SH, Garne JP, Lunge E. Over-diagnosis estimate from the Independent UK Panel on Breast Cancer Screening is based on unsuitable data. J Med Screen 2013;20:104–5.
16. Breast Cancer Surveillance Consortium. Breast Cancer Surveillance Consortium. Available at: https://www.bcsc-research.org/. Accessed July 09, 2020.
17. Hubbard RA, Kerlikowske K, Flowers CI, et al. Cumulative probability of false-positive recall or biopsy recommendation after 10 years of screening mammography: a cohort study. Ann Intern Med 2011;155:481–92.
18. Nelson HD, O'Meara ES, Kerlikowske K, et al. Factors associated with rates of false-positive and false-negative results from digital mammography screening: an analysis of registry data. Ann Intern Med 2016;164:226–35.
19. Tosteson AN, Fryback DG, Hammond CS, et al. Consequences of false-positive screening mammograms. JAMA Intern Med 2014;174(6):954–61.
20. Flores EJ, López D, Miles RC, et al. Impact of primary care physician interaction on longitudinal adherence to screening mammography across different racial/ethnic groups. J Am Coll Radiol 2019;16(7):908–14.
21. Berg WA. Benefits of screening mammography. JAMA 2010;303(2):168–9.
22. Siu AL, U.S. Preventive Services Task Force. Screening for Breast Cancer: U.S. Preventive Services Task Force Recommendation Statement. Ann Intern Med 2016;164(4):279–96 [Erratum appears in Ann Intern Med 2016;164(6):448].
23. Lee CH, Dershaw DD, Kopans D, et al. Breast cancer screening with imaging: recommendations from the Society of Breast Imaging and the ACR on the use of mammography, breast MRI, breast ultrasound, and other technologies for the detection of clinically occult breast cancer. J Am Coll Radiol 2010;7(1):18–27.
24. Expert Panel on Breast Imaging, Mainiero MB, Moy L, et al. ACR appropriateness criteria® breast cancer screening. J Am Coll Radiol 2017;14(11S):S383–90.
25. Miglioretti DL, Zhu W, Kerlikowske K, et al, Breast Cancer Surveillance Consortium. Breast tumor prognostic characteristics and biennial vs annual mammography, age, and menopausal status. JAMA Oncol 2015;1(8):1069–77.

26. Nelson HD, Tyne K, Naik A, et al, U.S. Preventive Services Task Force. Screening for breast cancer: an update for the U.S. Preventive Services Task Force. Ann Intern Med 2009;151(10):727–37. W237-42.

27. Wood ME, Rehman HT, Bedrosian I. Importance of family history and indications for genetic testing. Breast J 2020;26(1):100–4.

28. Lu KH, Wood ME, Daniels M, et al, American Society of Clinical Oncology. American Society of Clinical Oncology Expert Statement: collection and use of a cancer family history for oncology providers. J Clin Oncol 2014;32(8):833–40.

29. Lee C, McCaskill-Stevens W. Tomosynthesis mammographic Imaging Screening Trial (TMIST): an invitation and opportunity for the National Medical Association Community to shape the future of precision screening for breast cancer. J Natl Med Assoc 2020. https://doi.org/10.1016/j.jnma.2020.05.021. S0027-9684(20)30121-30128.

30. Lehman CD, Arao RF, Sprague BL, et al. National performance benchmarks for modern screening digital mammography: update from the breast cancer surveillance consortium. Radiology 2017;283(1):49–58.

31. Farber R, Houssami N, Wortley S, et al. Impact of full-field digital mammography versus film-screen mammography in population screening: a meta-analysis. J Natl Cancer Inst 2020. https://doi.org/10.1093/jnci/djaa080. djaa080.

32. Pisano ED, Hendrick RE, Yaffe MJ, et al. Diagnostic accuracy of digital versus film mammography: exploratory analysis of selected population subgroups in DMIST. Radiology 2008;246(2):376–83.

33. Marinovich ML, Hunter KE, Macaskill P, et al. Breast cancer screening using tomosynthesis or mammography: a meta-analysis of cancer detection and recall. J Natl Cancer Inst 2018;110(9):942–9.

34. Narayan AK, Elkin EB, Lehman CD, et al. Quantifying performance thresholds for recommending screening mammography: a revealed preference analysis of USPSTF guidelines. Breast Cancer Res Treat 2018;172(2):463–8.

35. Freer PE. Mammographic breast density: impact on breast cancer risk and implications for screening. Radiographics 2015;35(2):302–15.

36. Bakker MF, de Lange SV, Pijnappel RM, et al. Supplemental MRI screening for women with extremely dense breast tissue. N Engl J Med 2019;381(22):2091–102.

37. Comstock CE, Gatsonis C, Newstead GM, et al. Comparison of abbreviated breast MRI vs digital breast tomosynthesis for breast cancer detection among women with dense breasts undergoing screening. JAMA 2020;323(8):746–56 [Erratum appears in JAMA 2020;323(12):1194].

38. Burnside ES, Park JM, Fine JP, et al. The use of batch reading to improve the performance of screening mammography. AJR Am J Roentgenol 2005;185(3):790–6.

39. Froicu M, Mani KL, Coughlin B. Satisfaction with same-day-read baseline mammography. J Am Coll Radiol 2019;16(3):321–6.

40. Dontchos BN, Narayan AK, Seidler M, et al. Impact of a Same-Day Breast Biopsy Program on Disparities in Time to Biopsy. J Am Coll Radiol 2019;16(11):1554–60. https://doi.org/10.1016/j.jacr.2019.05.011. Epub 2019 May 29. PMID: 31152690.

41. Lehman CD, Yala A, Schuster T, et al. Mammographic breast density assessment using deep learning: clinical implementation. Radiology 2019;290(1):52–8.

Screening for Colorectal Cancer

Eric M. Montminy, MD[a], Albert Jang, MD[b], Michael Conner, MD[b],
Jordan J. Karlitz, MD[c,d],*

KEYWORDS

- Colorectal cancer • Screening • Epidemiology

KEY POINTS

- Colorectal cancer screening is available to providers in primary care settings to improve outcomes in colorectal cancer morbidity and mortality.
- Multiple colorectal cancer screening modalities are available to patients, with colonoscopy remaining the gold standard.
- Colorectal cancer screening rates are not optimized in many parts of the United States, with important barriers to screening including lack of health care provider recommendations and cost.
- It is important to identify higher-risk patients, including those with a family history of colorectal cancer or other cancers, so that earlier screening and possible genetic testing can be performed.

INTRODUCTION

Colorectal cancer (CRC) is the third most common cancer, excluding skin, to be diagnosed in men and women in the United States. The implementation of CRC screening for the detection of premalignant polyps has led to improvements in cancer incidence and survival. Several modalities for screening are available with varying degrees of sensitivity and specificity, but direct visualization with colonoscopy remains the gold standard for screening. This article provides context and guidance for clinicians preparing to discuss initiation of screening with patients.

[a] Division of Gastroenterology, Tulane University School of Medicine, 1430 Tulane Avenue, New Orleans, LA 70112, USA; [b] Department of Internal Medicine, Tulane University School of Medicine, 1430 Tulane Avenue, New Orleans, LA 70112, USA; [c] Southeast Louisiana Veterans Health Care System, Gastroenterology Section, 2400 Canal St, Medicine Service, Ste 3H, New Orleans, LA 70119, USA; [d] Division of Gastroenterology, Tulane University School of Medicine, New Orleans, LA 70112, USA
* Corresponding author.
E-mail address: jkarlitz@tulane.edu

Med Clin N Am 104 (2020) 1023–1036
https://doi.org/10.1016/j.mcna.2020.08.004
0025-7125/20/Published by Elsevier Inc.

medical.theclinics.com

BURDEN OF COLORECTAL CANCER IN UNITED STATES

The CRC mortality in the United States is currently the second highest of all cancers (after lung) for men and women combined. According to the National Cancer Institute, in 2016 the prevalence of CRC was estimated to be 1.3 million cases in the United States.[1] Current 2020 United States predictions estimate approximately 150,000 patients will be diagnosed with CRC, with more than 53,000 deaths.[2] Five-year survival rates range from 90% with localized disease to 14% with metastases, with overall survival rate at any stage of 65%. Lifetime risk of developing CRC is approximately 5%.[2]

Disparities between incidence and survival exist among different ethnic groups in the United States (**Fig. 1**).[2,3] Comparing ethnicities, African Americans consistently have significantly increased mortality and decreased 5-year survival. African Americans have CRC incidence rates of 53.8 per 100,000 for men and 39.9 per 100,000 for women, the highest incidence rates for any ethnic group.[4] White CRC incidence rates of 44.0 per 100,000 for men and 33.9 per 100,000 for women have been observed.[2] Hispanic Americans currently show lower incidences compared with white people: 40.8 per 100,000 for men and 28.7 per 100,000 for women.[2] Asian Americans continue to show the lowest incidence among all ethnic groups: 35.3 per 100,000 for men and 25.7 per 100,000 for women.[2] American Indian and Alaska Natives have a very high burden of disease, showing an incidence of 48.5 per 100,000 for men and 39.1 per 100,000 for women.[2]

Hispanic people are the fastest-growing minority population in the United States, and their population is younger than the average American population, so incidence rates are expected to increase in the upcoming decades.[5,6] Moreover, Hispanic people show higher mortalities from metastatic CRC compared with white people, and in turn, Hispanic people may show a higher mortality burden from CRC in the coming decades.[5,6]

Despite a lower incidence of CRC relative to other ethnicities, CRC is still the most common cancer diagnosed among Asian Americans.[7] Among east and southeast Asians, CRC screening rates are lower compared with African Americans and white people but higher compared with Hispanic people.[7] Importantly, wide variations in screening exist among individual Asian subgroups.[7]

The American Indian and Alaskan Native population also has CRC incidence and mortality that are higher than those of white people. Although incidence and mortality declined among white people in recent decades, it did not change for the American Indian and Alaskan Native population.[8] American Indian and Alaskan Native

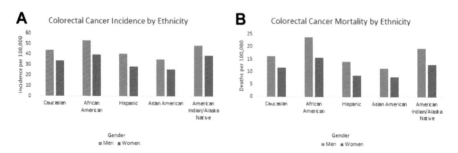

Fig. 1. CRC incidence (*A*) and mortality (*B*) rates in men and women by ethnicity, 2012 to 2017. African American men and women have the highest incidence and mortalities compared with other ethnicities. (*Adapted from* Siegel RL, Miller KD, Sauer AG, et al. Colorectal Cancer Statistics, 2020. CA Cancer J Clin. 2020; 70: 7-30. With permission.)

populations also have lower CRC screening rates compared with African Americans and white people.[9]

Regarding age, approximately 50% of all cases are diagnosed by age 65 years, and nearly 80% are diagnosed by age 80 years.[2] Recent attention has been directed toward so-called early-onset CRC.[2] Observations using Surveillance, Epidemiology, and End Results (SEER) analysis have shown acceleration of early-onset CRC incidence in patients aged 20 to 49 years over the last 3 decades.[2] Reasons for increasing early-onset CRC incidence are unclear at this time but may include alcohol consumption, diets consisting of red and processed meat, tobacco abuse, increasing obesity, and advanced endoscopic detection techniques.[10] It is thought that there is a potential underlying birth cohort effect associated with these increasing CRC rates, and increasing incidence has also been seen in 50 to 54-year-olds.[2] A recent study analyzing SEER data in 1-year age increments, as opposed to age range blocks, revealed a steep 46.1% incidence rate increase in CRCs from age 49 to 50 years, and 92.9% of these were invasive (beyond in situ stage).[11] These findings are consistent with a large undetected preclinical cancer burden ultimately diagnosed with screening at age 50 years, which is not reflected in observed SEER incidence rates.

NATURAL HISTORY OF COLORECTAL CANCER DEVELOPMENT

CRC is the umbrella term used for malignant neoplasms associated with various histologies throughout the colon and rectum. Among the various malignant neoplasms, almost all CRC is adenocarcinoma.[8] Adenocarcinomas develop from adenomas, which have varying degrees of dysplasia (potential to develop into an invasive malignancy).[12]

The progression of normal colorectal mucosa to adenoma to adenocarcinoma has been well defined. Several genetic mutations have been identified to initiate and promote the sequence of advancing dysplasia (**Fig. 2**). Most adenomatous polyps begin to develop from previously normal colorectal mucosa after expression of either an inherited or acquired mutation in the adenomatous polyposis coli gene (APC) and/or DNA mismatch repair gene (MMR). Early adenomas then typically progress to higher-risk adenomas if mutations such as K-Ras gene (KRAS) are expressed.

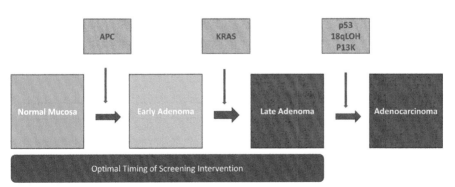

Fig. 2. Typical development of adenocarcinoma from adenoma. Note timing of each mutation along the progression of normal mucosa to adenocarcinoma. Ideally, CRC screening should be performed before the development of adenocarcinoma, when early and late adenomas can be detected and removed. APC, adenomatous polyposis coli; KRAS, K-Ras; PI3K, phosphatidylinositol 3 kinase.

Thereafter, loss of other apoptotic and cellular proliferation regulatory genes may accrue, leading to invasive adenocarcinomas.[12]

Adenomas have varying histologic classifications that hold different malignant potentials. Typical classifications of adenomas include a spectrum of tubular, tubulovillous, and villous histology depending on what percentage of each is visualized on pathology.[13] Tubular adenomas typically possess lower malignant potential, whereas villous adenomas hold higher malignant potential.[13] In general, polyps larger than 1 cm are associated with higher risk for malignancy compared with polyps less than 1 cm.[13] Importantly, all adenomas possess a degree of dysplasia and, in turn, a risk of malignant transformation over time.[13] If possible, adenomas should be removed when identified to minimize the chance of malignant transformation.

In addition, polyps can be defined by a sawtooth architecture visualized histologically with serration.[14] These polyps are often described endoscopically as flat (sessile) polyps and are often found within the right colon (ascending colon and cecum).[14] Depending on size, location, and exact histology, such polyps may be associated with various degrees of malignant potential. Specific guidelines are available focusing on the management and colonoscopy surveillance intervals for such lesions.[15]

COLORECTAL CANCER RISK FACTORS

Both modifiable and nonmodifiable risk factors for CRC have been established, and mitigating these risk factors plays an integral role in CRC prevention (**Table 1**). Modifiable risk factors such as tobacco and alcohol abuse, obesity, processed and red meats, and physical inactivity are abundant in the United States.[16] At the time of initiating CRC screening, modifiable risk factors should be discussed in order to further reduce CRC risk. Nonmodifiable CRC risks include aging, inflammatory bowel disease (ulcerative colitis or Crohn disease), prior abdominal radiation exposure, and family history of CRC or high-risk polyps.[16]

COLORECTAL CANCER RISK FACTORS: FAMILY HISTORY AND GENETIC SYNDROMES

Of the nonmodifiable risk factors for CRC, family history of CRC is significantly impactful. People with a first-degree relative (parent, sibling, or child) who have CRC have a 2 to 4 times risk of developing CRC themselves.[17] A family history of advanced colorectal polyps is also a significant, and underrecognized, CRC risk factor. This history

Table 1	
Modifiable and nonmodifiable risk factors associated with the development of colorectal cancer	
Risk Factors	
Modifiable	**Nonmodifiable**
Obesity	Aging
Physical inactivity	Inflammatory bowel disease
Tobacco abuse	Abdominal and pelvic radiation
Alcohol abuse	Hereditary CRC Syndromes
Diets high in red and	Family history of CRC or
processed meats	high-risk polyps
Cooking meats to	Personal history of
high temperatures	colorectal polyps
	Ethnicity
	Type 2 diabetes mellitus

includes any family history of a tubular adenoma greater than or equal to 1 cm and/or with villous features or high-grade dysplasia regardless of size. In addition, any family history of sessile serrated polyps greater than or equal to 1 cm or cytologic dysplasia and family history of traditional serrated adenomas should be discussed. First-degree relatives of patients with these advanced adenomas have significantly increased risk for CRC (1.68–3.80-fold increase) and advanced adenoma (6.05-fold increase).[18] It is important that providers ask patients not just about a family history of cancer but also about their family history of polyps so that proper risk stratification takes place. It is also recommended that, if an advanced polyp is diagnosed on colonoscopy, the provider who performed the colonoscopy should counsel the patient with the polyp that the patient's first-degree relatives are at increased risk and will need earlier screening (screening guidelines are discussed later).

People with a history of a mendelian cancer syndromes (such as Lynch syndrome) or polyposis syndromes (such as familial adenomatous polyposis or mutY homolog (MUTYH)-associated polyposis) have among the highest risk for CRC.[19] Mendelian CRC syndromes account for about 5% of CRC, with much higher percentages in patients with early-onset CRC.[20] Individuals that are carriers of the underlying genetic mutations can develop cancer at a much younger age than other high-risk groups and must initiate screening as early as their first decade of life depending on the syndrome and underlying mutation. The National Comprehensive Cancer Network (NCCN) "Genetic/Familial High-Risk Assessment: Colorectal" guidelines are an excellent resource that provide continually updated information on syndromic CRC, including information on genetic testing, diagnosis, and surveillance recommendations.[21] The guidelines also provide information on extracolonic cancers that have shown new associations with syndromes, such as breast and prostate cancer in Lynch syndrome.

A thorough family history should always be performed in order to identify patients that may require genetic testing. Knowledge of family history is also critical in order to determine timing of CRC screening in family members (how guidelines differ is discussed later) even if thresholds for need for germline testing are not met. A recent publication revealed that, in patients 40 to 49 years old with CRC, 1 in 4 met criteria for earlier screening based on family history and could have had their cancers detected earlier or prevented altogether if earlier screening had been initiated as per guidelines.[22]

Many of the tools focused on identifying Lynch syndrome are heavily weighted toward obtaining an accurate family history, such as the Prediction Model for MLH1, MSH2, MSH6, PMS2, and EPCAM Gene Mutations (PREMM5 Model).[20,a] This model is a particularly useful online tool in which basic information on personal and family history of cancer is entered into a Web site and a percentage chance of having an underlying Lynch syndrome mutation is quickly provided. A family history of extracolonic cancers may also indicate an underlying syndrome, and hence it is important for providers to ask patients about the patient's family history of all cancer types. For example, uterine cancer is the most common extracolonic cancer in Lynch syndrome, with up to 57% of patients developing uterine cancer depending on the underlying mutation.[21]

---

[a] The Bethesda guidelines, Amsterdam criteria, and PREMM5 are prediction models used to quantify an individual's risk for carrying a Lynch syndrome–associated mismatch repair gene and then decide whether further genetic testing is indicated.

Patients confirmed to be carriers of any of the mendelian CRC genes should be referred to a specialist in order to initiate screening at the appropriate age and determine intervals for follow-up examinations. Note that hereditary cancer syndromes are frequently under-recognized but carry substantial risk for both patients and family members. It is estimated that 1 in 279 people in the general population are Lynch syndrome carriers but many are unaware that they are carriers.[23] Even in young patients who have been diagnosed with CRC, diagnostic testing for Lynch syndrome is infrequently performed, placing patients and family members at high risk.[24]

It should also be noted that the NCCN guidelines currently recommend that all patients diagnosed with CRC, regardless of age, should undergo tumor testing with microsatellite instability or immunohistochemistry analysis as an initial screen for Lynch syndrome. For polyposis syndromes, it is important for providers to be mindful of the lifetime cumulative number of polyps (not just on a single colonoscopy), which may be overlooked, so that determination of the need for genetic testing can be made.

COLORECTAL CANCER SCREENING EFFECTIVENESS
Colonoscopy

Colonoscopy involves the use of a fiberoptic endoscope to examine the entire length of the colon in a sedated patient after bowel preparation. Of all screening modalities, colonoscopy has been shown to be the gold standard for detection and removal of premalignant colorectal polyps and detection of CRC.[25] Colonoscopy has been validated as an effective and superior CRC screening modality since the 1990s in both average-risk and high-risk patients. Extensive evidence from large randomized controlled trials such as the National Polyp Study Workgroup in 1993 studying colonoscopy with polypectomy in average-risk adults showed decreased incidence of CRC as high as 90% depending on location of cancer.[26] Advantages of colonoscopy include the highest sensitivity and specificity for detecting CRC and premalignant polyps compared with other screening modalities, as well as a potential 10-year screening interval in average-risk patients.[25] Disadvantages of colonoscopy include the need for bowel preparation and sedation as well as possible additional cost sharing not covered by commercial insurance or Medicare/Medicaid.[25] Although rare, colonoscopy carries procedural risks of mucosal injury such as laceration, bleeding, and perforation, as well as infection with instrumentation.

Quality measures for colonoscopy have been introduced to gives providers and patients perspective on screening performance. Metrics such as adenoma detection rate, adequacy of bowel preparation, and cecal withdrawal times have been introduced in order to improve the quality of colonoscopy and patient outcomes.[25] These individual metrics can be discussed with the provider who will be performing the procedure before screening to ensure a high-quality examination.

Stool-Based Screening

Fecal immunochemical testing (FIT) and guaiac fecal occult blood testing (gFOBT) are two stool-based CRC screening tests that are intended for outpatient CRC screening on an annual interval.[25] Both stool-based tests rely on detection of occult volumes of blood components taken up by stool as it passes over a friable cancer. FIT has shown higher CRC detection rates compared with gFOBT, and therefore FIT is primarily used.[27] Of marketed gFOBT kits, the American Cancer Society (ACS) only recommends using the newer, highly sensitivity guaiac test for CRC screening.[28]

FIT shows CRC screening sensitivity rates of approximately 80%, but detection of advanced adenomas is less than that of colonoscopy and has minimal sensitivity for sessile serrated polyps. At present, the United States Multi-Society Task Force[b] (USMSTF) labels FIT as an alternative tier 1 screening modality for patients opting not to undergo colonoscopy and willing to undergo yearly screening intervals.[25,c] Advantages of CRC screening with FIT center on decreased invasiveness and substantially less cost.[25] These advantages may be a factor for patients who are hesitant to undergo sedation or bowel preparation. Disadvantages include the need for yearly testing, higher false-positive rates compared with colonoscopy, and inability to intervene directly on precancerous lesions at time of screening.[25] Quality initiatives of FIT have primarily focused on improving access to FIT in the primary care setting and ensuring patients with positive FIT are promptly referred for colonoscopy.[25]

The more recently developed FIT-fecal DNA testing has been introduced as another alternative modality for CRC screening. FIT-fecal DNA testing incorporates detection of blood products and abnormal DNA genetic components such as KRAS mutations within stool into 1 test.[29] FIT-DNA testing is performed every 3 years as opposed to annually with traditional FIT. Advantages include increased sensitivity for cancers, advanced adenomas, and serrated polyps compared with FIT alone, although sensitivity is lower than that of colonoscopy.[30] According to the USMSTF, disadvantages primarily involve lower specificity rates (87% for FIT-DNA, 94% for FIT alone) compared with colonoscopy and FIT as well as higher cost.[25,31]

Computed Tomography Colonography (Virtual Colonoscopy)

Computed tomography (CT) colon imaging with air insufflation (known as CT colonography) has been used for CRC screening. CT colonography has been reported to detect CRC with sensitivities as high as 96%, although studies have largely been performed in symptomatic adults.[32] Prior comparisons of CT colonography with colonoscopy have shown CT colonography identifying precancerous adenomas at lower rates compared with colonoscopy.[33,34] CT colonography is associated with radiation exposure and the need for specific radiology facilities. It has been labeled a tier 2 CRC screening option by the USMSTF and may appeal to a niche of patients who are concerned about the risk of colonoscopy.[25] Like colonoscopy, CT colonography requires bowel preparation before an examination in order to optimize cancer detection. In addition, if a polyp is detected, colonoscopy is often recommended for direct visualization and removal.

Video Capsule Endoscopy

Video capsule endoscopy (VCE) involves swallowing a pill-shaped camera device that captures pictures of the intestinal mucosa throughout transit from mouth to anus after bowel preparation. With adequate bowel preparation, VCE has reached a sensitivity of 88% for adenomas larger than 6 mm but performed significantly worse for detection of serrated polyps.[25,35] VCE is not approved by the US Food and Drug Administration for average-risk CRC screening but may be used as an adjunct tool to visualize proximal colon lesions in patients with incomplete screening colonoscopy or patients who are not candidates for colonoscopy.[25]

---

[b] The USMSTF of CRC represents the American College of Gastroenterology (ACG), American Society of Gastrointestinal Endoscopy (ACGE), and American Gastroenterological Association (AGA).

[c] Currently the United States Preventive Services Task Force (USPSTF) does not tier screening modalities and instead highlights that there is convincing evidence that CRC screening substantially reduces deaths in patients 50 to 75 years old.[35]

Flexible Sigmoidoscopy

Flexible sigmoidoscopy is an endoscopic examination of the distal colon typically reaching as far as the splenic flexure. In the past, flexible sigmoidoscopy has been used as an effective CRC screening option for distal CRC; however, this modality has been largely replaced by colonoscopy because of the decreased ability of flexible sigmoidoscopy to detect proximal colon cancer.[25] Like colonoscopy, flexible sigmoidoscopy allows intervention on precancerous polyps at the time of screening and can be performed without sedation, if necessary.[25]

Septin 9 Assay

The Septin 9 assay is a serum-based CRC screening test that is intended to detect levels of Septin 9, a biomarker shed into the bloodstream after CRC development. Although approved for CRC screening, the Septin 9 assay shows markedly inferior sensitivity for the detection of CRC compared with other screening modalities. More recent pooled analyses observed sensitivities as high as 69% and specificity of 92% for CRC detection, but minimal to no adenoma sensitivity.[36]

HOW GUIDELINES DIFFER BETWEEN NATIONAL SOCIETIES' SCREENING RECOMMENDATIONS
American Cancer Society and United States Preventive Services Task Force

The ACS updated guidelines in 2018 to recommend initiating CRC screening in average-risk patients at 45 years old instead of 50 years old. Initiating earlier average-risk screening has been recommended based on increasing early-onset CRC incidence rates and modeling studies focused on life-years gained by initiating screening at 45 versus 50 years old.[37] ACS recommends screening should continue until 75 years old if the patient is in good health with a life expectancy more than 10 years.[37] The decision to continue past 75 years old and up until 85 years old should be based on patient preference, lack of previous screening history, and overall health.[25,37] The ACS recommends offering different screening options, including stool-based tests and structural examinations (such as colonoscopy) and performing the test that is most likely able to be completed.[28] Any abnormal screening test that is not an initial screening colonoscopy must be followed up with a diagnostic colonoscopy. The ACS screening approach is similar to the recommendation from the USPSTF, which recommends choosing a screening option based on patient preference and adherence, as well as medical contraindications and resources/availability.[38]

The United States Multi-Society Task Force on Colorectal Cancer

The USMSTF recommends initiating screening at 50 years old in average-risk individuals, with the exception of average-risk African Americans who should initiate screening at 45 years old. Based on the new ACS screening guidelines in 2018 recommending screening initiation at 45 years old, the USMSTF released a statement reporting that this change may improve early detection and prevention of CRC in younger individuals. The statement also reported that this change only addresses part of the increasing risk of CRC in younger individuals and that prompt assessment of symptoms consistent with CRC remains critical in persons less than 50 years of age.[39] The USMSTF shares similar guidelines to the ACS on screening discontinuation at 75 versus 85 years old.

In contrast with the USPSTF and ACS, the USMSTF recommends a sequential approach, in which health care providers offer patients preferred testing first and, if

Table 2
United States Multi-Society Task Force tier recommendation of screening modalities with respective screening intervals

Tier Recommendation	Screening Modality	Screening Interval
Tier 1	Colonoscopy	Every 10 y
	FIT	Annual
Tier 2	FIT-DNA	Every 3 y
	CT colonography	Every 5 y
	Flexible sigmoidoscopy	Every 5 y
Tier 3	VCE	Every 5 y

declined, offer the next highest-performance testing.[25] Stool-based testing and direct visualization are divided into tiers in order to follow the sequential approach (**Table 2**). Although the USMSTF still reports that the best test is the one that gets done, a tiered approach is recommended in order to have screening options with higher sensitivity and cost-effectiveness completed more frequently.[25] By following this approach and starting with tier 1, colonoscopy should be offered first, but, if refused, FIT is an appropriate second option. If both of these options are refused, the tiered system allows providers to offer the next highest-performing test by moving to tier 2 and then tier 3.

High-Risk Individuals

Most high-risk individuals should start CRC screening at an earlier age, ideally with colonoscopy.[37] Individuals with a family history of CRC or advanced adenomas, but no history of mendelian CRC syndromes (discussed earlier in relation to family history and genetic syndromes), should follow screening recommendations depending on the number of first-degree relatives and their respective ages of diagnosis. Per USMSTF guidelines, individuals with a single first-degree relative diagnosed with CRC or an advanced adenoma before age 60 years or 2 first-degree relatives diagnosed at any age should be screened with colonoscopy starting at age 40 years or 10 years earlier than the relative's diagnosis, whichever is earlier. Examinations can be repeated at 5-year intervals or possibly more frequently depending on findings. Individuals with a single first-degree relative diagnosed with CRC or an advanced adenoma at or after age 60 years can be offered average-risk screening options but beginning at age 40 years.[25]

COLORECTAL CANCER SCREENING IN THE UNITED STATES: HOW CAN IT BE IMPROVED?

Despite local and national initiatives, CRC screening rates among different communities generally are not optimal. At present, screening rates vary in patients aged 50 to 75 years depending on whether they seek screening through private insurance (72% screened), Medicare (62% screened), or a federally funded community clinic (44.1% screened).[40] The National Colorectal Cancer Roundtable (NCCRT) launched the 80% by 2018 initiative, and subsequently the 80% in Every Community initiative, which focus on improving national and individual community CRC screening rates to 80% of their respective populations. The NCCRT continually updates the progress of these initiatives in order to identify disparities in which resources can be focused, including low-income and rural populations and racial/ethnic minority communities, which can vary both between and within states. The lowest CRC screening rates have been observed in Latin-American, Native American, and Asian-American minority communities.[17] States such as Wyoming, Texas, and Nevada currently show some of the lowest percentages of state-wide populations undergoing CRC screening.[17] In response, the NCCRT has worked with national/local governments, academic institutions, cancer survivor groups, and insurance payers to identify and address screening barriers (**Box 1**). Barriers identified include financial cost of screening, lack of patients established with a primary care physician, so-called therapeutic inertia (ie, resistance to a clinical treatment by a patient or clinician), access to screening, and lack of screening navigators.[41] One of the most important barriers is lack of addressing CRC screening in the primary care setting. With further outreach, NCCRT hopes to reach 80% CRC screening rates in all communities. Clinicians and health care networks can find further tools and resources for improving CRC screening rates in each community through the NCCRT Internet-based platform: www.nccrt.org/resource-center.

KEY RECOMMENDATIONS FOR IMPLEMENTING SCREENING IN THE PRIMARY CARE SETTING
Establishing Patient Expectations

Patients approaching the timing of CRC screening should be adequately informed on expectations of screening goals and options. This discussion ideally should begin in the years leading up to the initiation of screening, because often there are delays between the time discussing CRC screening and the examination occurring. Asking questions such as, "What is your understanding of colorectal screening?" can elicit patient perspective to build on. Thorough discussions of family history of CRC or high-risk polyps can be discussed in the years leading up to screening initiation to determine the appropriate age to begin screening. Family history of CRC (and other types of cancer that may be associated with hereditary syndromes) and high-risk polyps is important to update with each health care maintenance visit because changes in family history can change the timing and interval of screening recommendations for the patient.

In addition, providers should discuss the importance of continued CRC screening during health care maintenance encounters in order to improve patient adherence to screening intervals. Providing easily accessible Web-based and print information on CRC screening to patients in an outpatient office can aid with directing patient attention toward different screening options and recommended screening intervals. Overall goals of screening expectations should be to provide patients with adequate

---

Box 1
Identified barriers to colorectal cancer screening

Lack of access to a primary care physician

Lack of provider recommendations for screening

Financial cost

Therapeutic Inertia

Lack of access to screening modalities

No access to screening navigators

resources to make informed decisions on screening in order to allow individualization of care.

Screening Availability and Access to Colonoscopy

Providers should understand which screening tests and referral centers are most accessible to patients before initiating CRC screening discussions. With the advent of outpatient endoscopy centers, access to screening colonoscopy and diagnostic colonoscopy if another screening test (eg, stool-based test, CT colonography) is positive has improved, but in some settings access to colonoscopy is still restricted. Patient navigator networks have been incorporated successfully in primary care settings and can be used to optimize access to screening modalities such as colonoscopy and referrals for expedited colonoscopy if another screening test is positive.[42]

Costs of Colorectal Cancer Screening

Commercial and government-provided insurance plans cover most CRC screening modalities. Patients should be provided an understanding of screening cost and potential for cost sharing. For example, health insurance plans established through the Patient Protection and Affordable Care Act removed cost sharing from polypectomy during screening colonoscopy. However, Medicare and Medicaid plans may require patients undergoing screening colonoscopy to participate with cost sharing if polypectomy is performed during the examination.[43] Ongoing federal legislation is being reviewed in order to address these cost-sharing measures.[44,45] It is beneficial for patients to have a discussion with insurance providers to understand payment issues associated with screening options.

DISCLOSURE

J.J. Karlitz serves as consultant to Exact Sciences Corporation as well as being a consultant and part of the speakers bureau for Myriad Genetics. Dr J.J. Karlitz has an equity position in Gastro Girl.

DISCLAIMER

The contents in this article do not necessarily reflect the views of the Department of Veterans Affairs or the US government.

REFERENCES

1. Surveillance, Epidemiology, and End results (SEER) Program. SEER*Stat Database: mortality-all COD, Aggregated with state, Total US (1969-2017) <Katrina/Rita population Adjustment>. National cancer Institute, Division of cancer Control and population Sciences, surveillance Research Program, cancer Statistics Branch; 2019; underlying mortality data provided. National Center for Health Statistics; 2019.

2. Siegel RL, Miller KD, Sauer AG, et al. Colorectal Cancer Statistics, 2020. CA Cancer J Clin 2020;70:7–30.

3. Montminy EM, Karlitz JJ, Landreneau SW. Progress of colorectal cancer screening in United States: past achievements and future challenges. Prev Med 2019;120:78–84.

4. DeSantis CE, Miller KD, Sauer AG, et al. Cancer Statistics for African Americans, 2019. CA Cancer J Clin 2019;69:211–33.

5. Hernandez-Nieto R, Gutierrez MC, Moreno-Fernandez F. Hispanic map of the United States 2017 2017. Available at: http://cervantesobservatorio.fas.harvard.edu/sites/default/files/hispanic_map_2017en.pdf. Accessed April 3, 2020.

6. Barzi A, Yang D, Mostofizadh S, et al. Trends in colorectal cancer mortality in hispanics: a SEER analysis. Oncotarget 2012;8:108771–7.

7. Hwang H. Colorectal cancer screening among Asian Americans. Asian Pac J Cancer Prev 2013;14:4025–32.

8. Fleming M, Ravula S, Tatishchev S, et al. Colorectal carcinoma: pathologic aspects. J Gastrointest Oncol 2012;3:153–73.

9. Johnson-Jennings MD, Tarraf W, Hill KX, et al. United States colorectal cancer screening practices among american indians/alaska natives, blacks, and non-hispanic whites in the New Millennium (2001 to 2010). Cancer 2014;120:3192–299.

10. Mauri G, Sartore-Bianchi A, Russo AG, et al. Early-onset colorectal cancer in young individuals. Mol Oncol 2019;13:109–31.

11. Abualkhair WH, Zhou M, Ahnen D, et al. Trends in incidence of early-onset colorectal cancer in the United States among those approaching screening age. JAMA Netw Open 2020;3:e1920407.

12. Carvalho B, Sillars-Hardebol AH, Postma C. Colorectal adenoma to carcinoma progression is accompanied by changes in gene expression associated with aging, chromosomal instability, and fatty acid metabolism. Cell Oncol (Dordr) 2012;35:53–63.

13. Calderwood AH, Lasser KE, Roy HK. Colon adenoma features and their impact on risk of future advanced adenomas and colorectal cancer. World J Gastrointest Oncol 2016;8:826–34.

14. Rex DK, Ahnen DJ, Baron JA, et al. Serrated lesions of the colorectum: review and recommendations from an expert panel. Am J Gastroenterol 2012;107:1315–30.

15. Lieberman DA, Rex DK, Winawer SJ, et al. Guidelines for colonoscopy surveillance after screening and polypectomy: a consensus update by the US multisociety task force on colorectal cancer. Gastroenterology 2012;143:844–57.

16. Johnson CM, Wei C, Ensor JE, et al. Meta-analyses of colorectal cancer risk factors. Cancer Causes Control 2013;24:1207–22.

17. American Cancer Society. Colorectal cancer facts & figures 2020-2022. Atlanta (GA): American Cancer Society; 2020.

18. Molmenti CL, Kolb JM, Karlitz JJ. Advanced colorectal polyps on colonoscopy: a trigger for earlier screening of family members. Am J Gastroenterol 2020;115:311–4.

19. Syngal S, Brand RE, Church JM. ACG clinical guideline: genetic testing and management of hereditary gastrointestinal cancer syndromes. Am J Gastroenterol 2015;110:223–63.

20. Tomlinson Ian. The mendelian colorectal cancer syndromes. Ann Clin Biochem 2015;52:690–2.

21. National Comprehensive Cancer Network. Genetic/Familial High-Risk Assessment: Colorectal. Available at: https://www.nccn.org/professionals/physician_gls/default.aspx#genetics_colon. Accessed June 14, 2020.

22. Gupta S, Bharti B, Ahnen DJ, et al. Potential impact of family history–based screening guidelines on the detection of early-onset colorectal cancer. Cancer 2020;126:3013–20.

23. Yurgelun MB, Hampel H. Recent advances in lynch syndrome: diagnosis, treatment, and cancer prevention. Am Soc Clin Oncol Educ Book 2018;38:101–9.

24. Karlitz JJ, Hsieh MC, Liu Y, et al. Population-based lynch syndrome screening by microsatellite instability in patients ≤50: prevalence, testing determinants, and result availability prior to colon surgery. Am J Gastroenterol 2015;110:944–58.

25. Rex DK, Boland R, Dominitz JA, et al. Colorectal cancer screening: recommendations for physicians and patients from the U.S. multi-society task force on colorectal cancer. Am J Gastroenterol 2017;112:1016–30.

26. Winawer SJ, Zauber AG, Ho MN, et al. Prevention of colorectal cancer by colonoscopic polypectomy. the national polyp study workgroup. N Engl J Med 1993; 329:1977–81.

27. Kupper BE, Junior SA, Nakagawa WT, et al. Comparison between an Immunochemical Fecal Occult Blood Test and a Guaiac Based Fecal Occult Blood Test in Detection of Adenomas and Colorectal Cancer. Appl Cancer Res 2018;38(5).

28. American Cancer Society. Colorectal cancer screening tests. 2018. Available at: https://www.cancer.org/cancer/colon-rectal-cancer/detection-diagnosis-staging/screening-tests-used.html. Accessed July 24,2020.

29. Imperiale TF, Ransohoff DF, Itzkowitz SH, et al. Multitarget stool DNA testing for colorectal-cancer screening. N Engl J Med 2014;370:1287–97.

30. Heigh RI, Yab TC, Taylor WR, et al. Detection of colorectal serrated polyps by stool DNA testing: comparison with fecal immunochemical testing for occult blood (FIT). PLoS One 2014;9:e85659.

31. Song LL, Li YM. Current noninvasive tests for colorectal cancer screening: An overview of colorectal cancer screening tests. World J Gastrointest Oncol 2016;8:793–800.

32. Pickhardt PJ, Hassan C, Halligan S, et al. Colorectal cancer: CT colonography and colonoscopy for detection—systemic review and meta-analysis. Radiology 2011;259:393–405.

33. Weinberg DS, Pickhardt PJ, Bruining DH, et al. Computed tomography colonography vs colonoscopy for colorectal cancer surveillance after surgery. Gastroenterology 2018;154:927–34.

34. Duarte RB, Bernardo WM, Sakai CM, et al. Computed tomography colonography versus colonoscopy for the diagnosis of colorectal cancer: a systemic review and meta-analysis. Ther Clin Risk Manag 2018;14:349–60.

35. Rex DK, Adler SN, Aisenberg J, et al. Accuracy of capsule colonoscopy in detecting colorectal polyps in a screening population. Gastroenterology 2015; 148:948–57.

36. Hariharan R, Jenkins M. Utility of the methylated SEPT9 test for the early detection of colorectal cancer: a systematic review and meta-analysis of diagnostic test accuracy. BMJ Open Gastroenterol 2020;7:e000355.

37. American Cancer Society Guideline for Colorectal Cancer Screening. American Cancer Society. Available at: https://www.cancer.org/cancer/colon-rectal-cancer/detection-diagnosis-staging/acs-recommendations.html. Accessed April 2, 2020.

38. United States Preventive Services Task Force. Screening for Colorectal Cancer. US Preventive Services Task Force Recommendation Statement. JAMA 2016; 315(23):2564–75.

39. American Gastroenterological Association. Statement from the U.S. Multisociety Task Force on Colorectal Cancer. 2018. Available at: https://www.gastro.org/press-release/statement-from-the-u-s-multisociety-task-force-on-colorectal-cancer. Accessed May 5, 2020.

40. National Colorectal Cancer Roundtable. Colorectal Cancer Screening Rates. Available at: https://nccrt.org/data-progress/#:~:text=The%20UDS%20CRC%

20screening%20rate,exceeded%20an%2080%25%20screening%20rate.   Accessed June 1, 2020.

41. National Colorectal Cancer Round Table. Colorectal cancer screening data set update: how are we doing on our efforts to reach 80%?. 2019. Available at: https://nccrt.org/resource/colorectal-cancer-screening-data-set-update-how-are-we-doing-on-our-efforts-to-reach-80-january-28-2019/. Accessed June 1, 2020.

42. Escoffery C, Fernandez ME, Vernon SW, et al. Patient navigation in a colorectal cancer screening program. J Public Health Manag Pract 2015;21:433–40.

43. Howard DH, Guy GP, Ekwueme DU. Eliminating cost-sharing requirements for colon cancer screening in medicare. Cancer 2014;120:3850–2.

44. Removing Barriers to Colorectal Screening Act of 2015, H.R. 1220, 114th Congress 2015. Print.

45. SCREEN Act of 2015, H.R. 2035, 114th Congress 2015. Print.

Screening for Lung Cancer

Thomas Houston, MD*

KEYWORDS

- Lung cancer screening • Low-dose CT lung screening • Shared decision making
- Smoking cessation

KEY POINTS

- Lung cancer screening is the latest intervention designed to mitigate morbidity and mortality from cancer.
- This article briefly summarizes the history of lung cancer screening, its acceptance by primary care clinicians, elements of the intervention that are underutilized (smoking cessation and shared decision making), and integration of lung cancer screening into practice.
- Primary care physician practices related to low-dose computerized tomography have evolved slowly, and its uptake in their clinical practice has been low.
- Barriers to implementation of lung cancer screening in primary care include unfamiliarity with indications for screening, time constraints, competing health priorities, and questions about coverage.
- Both smoking cessation and shared decision making are integral to lung cancer screening, and are necessary components in its implementation.
- Gaps persist in creating a systematic approach to lung cancer screening in primary care practice; approaches to integrate lung cancer screening protocols are discussed.

INTRODUCTION

Lung cancer screening is the latest intervention designed to mitigate morbidity and mortality from cancer. This article briefly summarizes the history of lung cancer screening, its acceptance by primary care clinicians, elements of the intervention that are underutilized (smoking cessation and shared decision making [SDM]), and integration of lung cancer screening into practice.

To begin this discussion of lung cancer screening, the characteristics of a good cancer screening program as defined by Miser[1] set the stage:

"The cancer sought should be an important health problem. The prevalence of the cancer should be high enough to justify screening. The natural history of the cancer, including development from latent to declared disease, should be adequately

Department of Family Medicine, The Ohio State University College of Medicine, Columbus, OH, USA
* 4867 Calloway Court, Dublin, OH 43017.
E-mail address: tphdoc@aol.com

Med Clin N Am 104 (2020) 1037–1050
https://doi.org/10.1016/j.mcna.2020.08.005
0025-7125/20/© 2020 Elsevier Inc. All rights reserved.

understood. There should be a recognizable latent (asymptomatic) or early symptomatic stage in which detection is possible. Facilities for screening, diagnosis, and treatment should be available. There should be a suitable test or examination that is sufficiently sensitive to detect disease during the asymptomatic period but sufficiently specific to minimize false-positive results. The test should be acceptable to patients. Patients should be willing to agree to further evaluation of positive screening tests and follow through with treatment if cancer is diagnosed. There should be an accepted treatment for individuals with the newly diagnosed cancer, with outcomes improved by therapy during the asymptomatic period. There should be an agreed-on policy concerning whom to treat as patients. The cost of screening, diagnosis, and treatment should be balanced economically in relation to possible expenditure on medical care as a whole."

EVIDENCE FOR LUNG CANCER SCREENING

Lung cancer remains the leading cause of cancer death for both sexes in the United States; among men, it became the leading cause of cancer mortality in the mid-1950s, and in 1987 it overtook breast cancer to become the leading cancer killer among American women as well. Although smoking is the chief cause of lung cancer, other risk factors include exposure to secondhand smoke, occupational carcinogens, radon exposure, and family history. Despite reductions in lung cancer mortality of 51% among men since 1990 and 26% among women since 2002, the American Cancer Society (ACS) estimates that 135,720 lung cancer deaths will occur in the United States in 2020.[2] Most patients are not diagnosed until they are symptomatic and are found to have stage III or stage IV cancer, with 5-year survival rates of 16% and 4%, respectively.[3]

Because of the high mortality and difficulty in detecting lung cancer at early stages when surgery might be curative, there has long been interest in attempting early detection through screening, first with chest radiography and, beginning in the 1990s, with chest low-dose computed tomography (LDCT) scanning. Chest radiography was the subject of 3 US trials supported by the National Cancer Institute (NCI) in the 1970s, with studies at Memorial Sloan-Kettering, Johns Hopkins, and the Mayo Clinic. The Sloan-Kettering and Johns Hopkins trials added sputum cytology every 4 months to an annual chest radiograph and compared that with annual chest radiograph alone; the Mayo trial compared annual chest radiograph and sputum cytology every 3 months. The Memorial Sloan-Kettering and Johns Hopkins studies showed no difference in mortality rate by adding sputum cytology to annual chest radiograph. The Mayo Clinic study did not show a difference in mortality between groups or a shift toward detection of earlier-stage cancers and lacked sufficient power to detect a mortality advantage.[4,5]

Based on the finding from the NCI trials, in 1980 the ACS changed policy that had favored chest radiography as a tool for screening asymptomatic patients for lung cancer, recommended against any mass screening tests for early detection of lung cancer,[6] and began to emphasize prevention and tobacco cessation. They did continue to support chest radiographs for heavy smokers and asbestos workers, however. In a commentary published in *American Family Physician* later that year, the American Academy of Family Physicians (AAFP) described the changes in the ACS cancer screening recommendations as being "greeted cautiously" by the medical community and noted that the lung cancer recommendations had received the most negative reaction.[7] Physician behavior seemed hard to change—ACS surveys of cancer screening in 1984[8] and 1989[9] found 44% of primary care physicians (PCPs) in both surveys ordering chest radiographs for screening asymptomatic patients for lung cancer, well after the ACS and others had advised against its use.

A larger trial examining chest radiograph in lung cancer screening, the Prostate, Lung, Colorectal and Ovarian randomized trial, randomized 154,901 individuals either to annual chest radiograph or usual care, with sufficient power to detect a 10% difference in lung cancer mortality between intervention and control groups. Men and women at 10 centers were seen between 1993 and 2001. There was no eligibility requirement concerning smoking. The intervention group had a baseline chest radiograph and annual radiographs for 3 more years. There was no effects on cumulative lung cancer mortality over the 13 years of observation in the trial or stage shift in lung cancer at diagnosis. A subanalysis of patients who would have been candidates for the National Lung Screening Trial (NLST), which compared chest radiograph with LDCT scan, also found no difference between groups.[10]

In the early 1990s, studies began using LDCT scan as a modality for lung cancer screening. Studies in Japan[11] and the United States began in 1993[12] and were followed with studies in Europe.[13–15] The largest of the early US studies was the Early Lung Cancer Action Project, which enrolled 1000 high-risk patients (age 60 and older with at least 10 pack-year history of smoking) and found 27 to have cancer on enrollment, with only 7 of these seen on chest radiograph. At surgery, 85% of the tumors were stage 1A.[12]

Subsequent single-arm trials in Europe, Japan, and the United States affirmed that LDCT showed superiority over chest radiograph for lung cancer screening,[16–22] finding approximately 4 times more tumors than chest radiograph but did not show that screening saved lives. Subsequently, NLST and other randomized controlled trials provided unambiguous evidence of benefit of LDCT in reducing lung cancer mortality.

The NLST, published in 2011, enrolled 53,454 participants over 5 years. Individuals were between ages 55 and 74 with a 30 pack-year history of smoking, and LDCT was compared with chest radiograph using annual examination for 3 years. Median follow-up time was 5.6 years.[23] A total of 1060 lung cancers were found in the LDCT arm, compared with 941 in the chest radiograph group. Almost twice as many early-stage cancers were diagnosed with LDCT compared with chest radiograph (40% vs 21%, respectively). There was a 20% relative reduction in lung cancer mortality in the LDCT group; the number needed to screen to prevent 1 death was 320. This was the first trial to show a reduction in lung cancer–specific mortality through LDCT screening.[23]

Despite criticism about its false-positive tests, cost, overdiagnosis, and patient anxiety, the NLST spurred the adoption of lung cancer screening guidelines, most of which mirrored its study parameters. The first of these medical society guidelines was published in 2012, when Wood and colleagues[24] wrote the Clinical Guidelines in Oncology for Lung Cancer Screening for the National Comprehensive Cancer Network (NCCN), which have been updated annually. The NCCN agrees with the NLST/US Preventive Services Task Force (USPSTF) criteria and has issued 1 recommendation for LDCT screening that has the same smoking history criteria but also points out that lung cancer risk is not confined to cigarette smoking and has issued a companion guideline that includes other factors, such as radon exposure, occupational exposure to carcinogens, family history of lung cancer, and a personal history of cancer or chronic lung disease. This alternative guideline, which has become known as NCCN-2, targets adults with the presence of at least 1 of these additional risk factors, combined with a 20 pack-year smoking history (instead of 30), and expanded age criteria ($\geq$50 years and >77 years). Adults with a less intense smoking history and none of the other listed risk factors are classified as lower risk, and LDCT screening for lung cancer is not recommended.

Early in 2013, the ACS updated its lung cancer screening guideline and recommended the NLST eligibility criteria, similar to the NCCN,[24] emphasizing that clinicians with access to high-volume, high-quality lung cancer screening and treatment centers should initiate a discussion about annual LDCT screening for lung cancer with apparently healthy patients aged 55 years to 74 years who have at least a 30-pack-year smoking history and who currently smoke or have quit within the past 15 years.[25] Later in 2013, the USPSTF reviewed the NLST data and in 2013 issued a grade B recommendation supporting annual lung cancer screening with LDCT for asymptomatic individuals 55 years to 80 years of age with a 30 pack-year history of smoking who currently smoke or have quit within the past 15 years. The USPSTF further stressed that patients should be healthy enough to undergo lung surgery and be willing to undergo potentially curative treatment.[26] Since the USPSTF gave LDCT screening for lung cancer a B rating, provisions in the Patient Protection and Affordable Coverage Act require private insurance carriers to provide coverage for lung cancer screening without deductible or copay when patients meet the USPSTF criteria for screening.[27]

After publication of the NLST and the USPSTF recommendations, several other medical societies and health groups issued guidelines regarding lung cancer screening, most of which adhere closely to the USPSTF recommendations. **Table 1** summarizes the major medical society recommendations.

The AAFP reviewed the USPSTF recommendation in 2013 and issued a grade I recommendation (insufficient evidence to recommend either for or against

Table 1
Eligibility criteria for lung cancer screening with low-dose computed tomography

Organization	Age (y)	Smoking History (Pack-Years)	Years Since Quitting Smoking	Other
CMS	55–77	≥30	<15	—
USPSTF	55–80	≥30	<15	—
American Association for Thoracic Surgery				
Tier 1	55–79	≥30	—	Additional risk factor[a]
Tier 2	≥50	≥20	—	Lung cancer survivor >5 y
ACCP	55–77	≥30	<15	—
ACS	55–74	≥30	<15	—
NCCN				
Group 1	55–77	≥30	<15	—
Group 2	≥50	≥20	—	At least 1 additional risk factor[b]

Definition: 1 pack-year, having smoked an average of 1 pack of cigarettes per day for 1 y.
[a] Additional risk factors for lung cancer defined by the American Association for Thoracic Surgery include chronic obstructive pulmonary disease, environmental and occupational exposures, any prior cancer or thoracic radiation, and genetic or family history.
[b] Additional risk factors for lung cancer defined by NCCN include cancer history, lung disease history, family history of lung cancer, radon exposure, and occupational exposure.
Adapted from Fintelmann FJ, Gottmukkala RV, McDermott S, et al. Lung Cancer Screening: Why, When and How? Radiology Clinics of North America. 2017;55(6): p.1165; with permission.

screening).[28] This was based on concerns that the USPSTF decision was made chiefly from the findings of a single study, the NLST, which was not replicated in community settings and had only 3 annual computed tomography (CT) scans in the study. Cost, the need for SDM (USPSTF had not specified this intervention), the potential for radiation exposure, and the problems of potential harms from diagnostic follow-up of positive findings also were of concern to AAFP.

The Centers for Medicare and Medicaid Services (CMS) announced in 2015[29] that it would cover lung cancer screening services for patients ages 55 to 77 who met the other USPSTF metrics, with several provisions. The provider must engage the patient in an SDM encounter, discussing the risks and benefits of lung cancer screening, using decision aids that help the patient understand issues, such as radiation exposure, false-positive findings, the potential for follow-up diagnostic procedures, and the need for annual screening examinations. CMS also mandated that clinicians must offer smoking cessation services for patients who smoke.

In early 2020, the long-awaited results of the Dutch-Belgian Nederlands-Luvens Longkanker Screenings Onderzoek (NELSON) trial was published.[30] This trial recruited study subjects from 2000 to 2004, and enrolled 13,195 men and 2594 women randomized to undergo low-dose, volumetric LDCT scanning with baseline and 1-year, 3-year, and 5.5-year repeat scans versus no scanning. There was a shift toward earlier-stage diagnosis in the LDCT arm, and, at 10 years' follow-up, lung cancer mortality was 24% lower in men and 33% lower in women than the control group, thus confirming the major findings of the NLST. Use of node volume measurement and the doubling time of node volume likely resulted in higher sensitivity (93.5% vs 92.5%, respectively) and specificity (98.3% vs 73.4%, respectively) than the NLST.[30] Editorials accompanying publication of the NELSON trial stated emphatically that the efficacy of LDCT screening for lung cancer has clearly been affirmed.[31,32]

Although progress has been made in establishing lung cancer screening with LDCT through clinical trials and publication of professional society guidelines, uptake of lung cancer screening in clinical practice has been sluggish at best, and implementation of screening guidelines is inconsistent. Richards and colleagues[33] at the Centers for Disease Control and Prevention (CDC) analyzed the 2010 and 2015 National Health Interview Survey data, finding that in 2015 only 4.4% of patients eligible for lung cancer screening reported receiving an LDCT scans. Surprisingly, 8.5% of adults eligible for LDCT screening received a chest radiograph instead, and an estimated 1.8 million people not meeting USPSTF criteria inappropriately received an LDCT.[33] If lung cancer screening is to become as well integrated into practice as are more accepted programs, such as screening for breast or colorectal cancer, a variety of steps need to be undertaken through education and changes in practice patterns. Surveys of PCP attitudes and implementation of lung cancer screening reveals that lack of knowledge about screening guidelines and their implementation is a key barrier.[34] In addition, physicians identify several challenges with screening that include lack of time, patients with competing clinical priorities and health concerns, prior authorization and other insurance barriers, reimbursement, and uncertainty about referral protocols.

PRIMARY CARE PHYSICIAN ATTITUDES TOWARD LOW-DOSE COMPUTED TOMOGRAPHY SCREENING

PCP knowledge, attitudes, and practices related to LDCT screening for lung cancer have evolved slowly, but 9 years after publication of the NLST findings and 7 years since endorsement of LDCT screening by guideline-issuing organizations, surveys of PCPs still do not reveal a predominate readiness to implement LDCT screening for early lung cancer detection.

Lung cancer screening practices among PCPs were examined in a national survey published in 2012 before guidelines were issued by national authorities[35]; 25% of surveyed PCP believed that LDCT screening guidelines had been issued. More PCPs believed that LDCT was effective at screening than chest radiograph; few believed sputum cytology was useful. More believed screening was useful in current smokers, contrasted with former smokers. A substantial 34% thought LDCT would be useful in never-smokers. In the past year, 38% had ordered no lung cancer screening tests, 55% had ordered chest radiograph, 22% had ordered LDCT, and fewer than 5% had ordered sputum cytology. PCP were more likely to have ordered lung cancer screening tests if they (1) believed that expert groups recommend lung cancer screening or that lung cancer screening was effective; (2) if they would recommend screening for asymptomatic patients, including patients without substantial smoking exposure; and (3) if their patients had asked them about screening. The investigators were concerned about inappropriate screening by PCPs and overuse of technology that at the time was still unproved.[35]

Hoffman and colleagues[36] reported results of semistructured interviews with 10 PCPs in New Mexico in 2014, and found that both chest radiograph and LDCT scanning were being used for lung cancer screening. Several of those interviewed were not aware of the NLST results or other national recommendations. Respondents were skeptical about the false-positive rate, the number needed to screen to prevent 1 death, and the small proportion of minority participants in NLST. There was doubt about whether infrastructure was sufficient for screening and concerns about access and cost. The perceived complexity of conducting SDM discussions was perceived as another barrier. The investigators concluded that provider/patient education about lung cancer screening was needed and recommended support for informed decision making and initiatives to ensure that high-quality screening could be delivered in community practice, given the rural nature of the state.

Ersek and colleagues[37] conducted a 2015 survey of family physicians in South Carolina. Most had incorrect knowledge about which organizations recommended lung cancer screening—only 40% knew the USPSTF recommended LDCT screening. Many PCP continued to recommend chest radiograph for lung cancer screening. Most felt that LDCT screening increased the odds of detecting disease at earlier stages (98%) and that the benefits outweighed the harms (75%); however, paradoxically, only 40% thought screening reduced mortality. Concerns included unnecessary procedures (88%), patient stress/anxiety (52%), and radiation exposure (50%). Only 31% knew that Medicare covered LDCT screening. Most PCP reported that they discussed the risks/benefits of screening with their patients in some capacity (76%); however, more than 50% reported making 1 or no screening recommendations in the past year.

A national survey in 2016 to 2017 examined PCPs' knowledge, attitudes, referral practices, and associated barriers regarding LDCT screening.[38] More than half of the respondents correctly reported that the USPSTF recommends LDCT screening for high-risk patients. Although 75% agreed that the benefits of LDCT screening outweighed the risks, fewer agreed that there was substantial evidence that screening reduces mortality (50%). The most commonly reported barriers to ordering screening included prior authorization requirements (57%), lack of insurance coverage (53%), and coverage denials (31%). The most frequently cited barrier to conducting SDM was patients' competing health priorities (42%). Clinical practice and policy changes were suggested by the investigators as ways to engage more patients in screening discussions.

A 2017 survey found PCPs less confident than subspecialists in identifying patients who were candidates for lung cancer screening.[39] They were less comfortable than subspecialists in counseling patients about screening and reported inadequate time for counseling/screening activities. Despite these barriers, PCPs were equally likely to order lung cancer screening in their practice as subspecialists, likely because they were aware of USPSTF guidelines and were inclined to follow them. This study suggested the need for improving education for physicians, especially PCPs, related to lung cancer screening and the counseling that is involved.

Lewis and colleagues[34] found in a 2019 survey of academic and Veterans Affairs physicians in Nashville that 62% had low knowledge of lung cancer screening guidelines and 59% reported ordering LDCT screening. Referring provider screening was proportional to their knowledge of the guidelines; both physician education and system-level changes to support screening were suggested.

Although the uptake of lung cancer screening has been quite low, a 2020 CDC report[40] on a 10-state survey conducted in 2017 found that 12.5% of patients meeting the USPSTF screening criteria reported having received a screening LDCT scan, representing a sizable increase compared with earlier reports.[40–42] As in the Lewis and colleagues[34] survey, the CDC investigators recommended provider education and decision support tools to help increase screening. More educational opportunities for PCPs related to lung cancer screening recently have emerged, notably, the LuCa National Training Network online course, available without cost at https://www.lucatraining.org/.

IMPLEMENTATION OF LUNG CANCER SCREENING IN PRIMARY CARE PRACTICE

Despite the broad support for lung cancer screening by multiple organizations, LDCT screening continues to be underutilized in primary care. A recent survey confirmed that PCP are unfamiliar with the indications for lung cancer screening and have problems identifying eligible patients, a problem complicated by electronic medical record (EMR) deficiencies.[43] Other gaps include time constraints, competing health priorities, issues with insurance coverage, and patient comorbidities.[43,44] In addition, both smoking cessation and an SDM conversation with patients are required by CMS for reimbursement of lung cancer screening interventions. A brief overview of these aspects of lung cancer screening implementation may be useful.

SMOKING CESSATION

Because half of persons presenting for lung cancer screening still smoke cigarettes, the CMS mandate for smoking cessation interventions during the screening process presents an opportunity to deliver another life-saving clinical service. All of the professional societies that have developed lung cancer screening guidelines agree that lung cancer screening is not a substitute for smoking cessation interventions; thus, the CMS mandate is a reminder that tobacco treatment should be a standard of care for any current smoker, regardless of whether they quality for lung cancer screening or are age 65 and older. In the 2020 US Surgeon General report, "Smoking Cessation," lung cancer screening is listed among 2 "life events" that can trigger smoking cessation attempts, uptake of smoking cessation services, and smoking cessation.[45] The report further suggests that integration of smoking cessation services into lung cancer screening programs may increase smoking cessation.

A recent study of physician perceptions of lung cancer screening as a teachable moment for cessation found mixed views.[46] Some thought that the lung cancer screening discussion was a good opportunity to motivate patients to attempt cessation, whereas others did not think that lung cancer screening would motivate patients. Most physicians did believe that receiving screening results could affect patients' motivation to stop smoking; however, some physicians thought that a negative report would lead to a laissez-faire attitude and perpetuation of current smoking patterns.

Physicians often saw the smoking cessation intervention as being a different event than the SDM discussion and failed to integrate cessation into lung cancer screening. Lack of time, limited resources, and knowledge gaps contributed to missed opportunities in integrating smoking cessation into the lung cancer screening visit.

In the same study, many patients reported that the lung cancer screening experience triggered a strong emotional response, leading them to rethink their health priorities, and motivated them to consider smoking cessation. Some patients, however, reported that other life stressors prevailed and that they would continue to smoke.

The Association for Treatment of Tobacco Use and Dependence (ATTUD) and the Society for Research on Nicotine and Tobacco published a guideline for pairing lung cancer screening services and smoking cessation in 2016.[47] The guideline points out that the population being screened is, by and large, motivated to stop smoking and that pairing evidence-based smoking cessation methods with lung cancer screening is likely to have the potential to increase smoking cessation attempts, although data are limited (but promising) about the response of patients to these interventions.

The guideline summarizes the evidence for smoking cessation treatment in patients 55 to 77 years of age, including the 5 As approach to cessation (ask patients about whether they smoke; advise smokers to quit; assess willingness to quit at that time; assist them in quitting with practical counseling, a supportive clinical environment, links to supplemental support, and medication; and arrange for follow-up contact with smokers making a quit plan). The guideline discussed the use of motivational interviewing for patients who resist cessation interventions and the potential for smoking reduction as an interim step.

Specific resources for this population of older smokers were reviewed. Recommendations include

1. Encourage smokers who present for lung cancer screening to stop at each visit in the screening process, regardless of the screening result. Reinforcement of the message by different providers during the screening process may strengthen the intervention.
2. Provide patients with access to evidence-based behavioral counseling and pharmacotherapy for smoking cessation. These services could be provided by referring physicians, cessation clinics at the screening center, referral to tobacco treatment services, and/or the national tobacco cessation quitline (1–800-QUIT NOW).
3. Arrange follow-up through the referring provider or screening service to support cessation attempts.
4. For patients unwilling to make a quit attempt or reduce tobacco use, provide motivation with the 5 relevance, risks, rewards, roadblocks, and repetition (Rs) behavioral intervention.

The ATTUD guideline calls for further research into the optimal intensity and timing of cessation interventions in the context of lung cancer screening, the optimal delivery mode, the potential adverse effects of screening on tobacco cessation motivation, barriers to clinician implementation of cessation services within the context of lung cancer screening, and the educational needs of clinicians who could provide cessation services.

SHARED DECISION MAKING

As discussed previously, SDM has been mandated by CMS as a necessary component of the lung cancer screening encounter, and lung cancer screening is the only imaging or cancer screening intervention with this requirement. SDM is a patient-centered activity that ideally empowers individuals to take part in their care, assuming that when provided with good information, patients will be able to ask questions and provide their input into decisions about their care that align with their values and circumstances. Having taken part in SDM, clinicians should be more informed as well, providing services that are based on patient preferences and goals. If patients understand the benefits and risks of a procedure, SDM allows patients to actively assist in decisions regarding their care.[48] As with offering tobacco cessation services, this component of lung cancer screening often is not performed in a systematic, integrated way.[49,50]

Lowenstein and colleagues'[50] review of SDM in lung cancer screening points out that multiple components exist in SDM encounters:

- Discussion of the benefits of lung cancer screening, including the potential for early detection of disease, reduction in treatment morbidity comparing early-stage versus late-stage therapy, and possible reduction in mortality
- Discussion of the risks involved in screening, including the false-positive rate; risk of follow-up testing and procedures, although low; the possibility of overdiagnosis; and the risk of radiation
- The need to undergo annual LDCT until the patient no longer meets screening criteria
- Discussion of patient comorbidities
- Discussion of the patient's ability and willingness to undergo treatment
- Discussion of smoking cessation, if applicable

CMS requires the use of decision aids in the SDM discussion. These tools are meant to improve clinician-patient discussions and enhance patient knowledge. Decision aids provide information about lung cancer, the screening process, the benefits and risks of screening, and smoking cessation. Several decision aids have been developed and are discussed in detail by Lowenstein and colleagues.[50]

Implementation of SDM has been difficult to integrate into lung cancer screening visits. As an example, a report in 2020 from an academic medical center revealed that in interviews approximately 6 months after a lung cancer screening encounter, 85% of patients (n = 39) who completed screening and 89% of patients (n = 30) who declined screening could not recall having used a decision aid during the SDM conversation with the provider. Although 62% of patients who completed screening recalled that an SDM conversation had taken place, only 39% of patients who declined undergoing screening thought so. In reviewing the charts of all the patients in the survey, none had any documentation of the SDM conversation in the record. As with other screening measures, physicians cite several familiar reasons why they do not perform SDM, including lack of time, training, inadequate support, and lack of decision aids.[48]

Where and when should the SDM encounter occur? CMS reimburses clinicians for a separate SDM visit apart from the screening encounter itself, allowing for PCP to integrate SDM for lung cancer screening into routine clinical care before the referral. Another option is having the SDM encounter at the screening center. The provider may bill for the lung cancer screening SDM visit with the screening code G0296, defined as a counseling visit to discuss need for lung cancer screening using LDCT scanning (the service is for eligibility determination and SDM). The SDM conversation is not limited to physicians but can be carried out by other members of the health care team. The nurse navigator or another dedicated clinician could take on this role at the screening center, freeing up the physician for other responsibilities and giving more time for the SDM encounter.

The Agency for Healthcare Research and Quality (AHRQ) has developed tools to assist clinicians in assisting with improved SDM encounters. "Lung Cancer Screening Tools for Patients and Clinicians" contains a decision aid for patients to be reviewed before the SDM visit, a decision tool for patients and clinicians to be used for SDM, a lung cancer screening summary guide for primary care clinicians, and a checklist for clinicians that summarizes all the necessary components of lung cancer screening and decision making that allow the encounters to be covered as a preventive service visit under Medicare. The AHRQ tools can be found at https://effectivehealthcare.ahrq.gov/decision-aids/lung-cancer-screening/home.html.

Another summary resource on lung cancer screening and SDM has been developed by the American Thoracic Society, the American Lung Association, and Lung Force, and is available at https://www.lungcancerscreeningguide.org/shared-decision-making/shared-decision-making-resources/.

IMPLEMENTING LUNG CANCER SCREENING PROGRAMS

Particularly in nonacademic health centers, there is a need to create an integrated, systematic approach to lung cancer screening. The American College of Chest Physicians (ACCP) and the American Thoracic Society have developed a policy statement about implementation of lung cancer screening programs.[51] Bernstein and colleagues[52] described the creation of a lung cancer screening program in a nonacademic hospital system and point out several issues to be considered. First, the need for key physician leadership (in their experience, from pulmonary, radiology, and thoracic surgery physicians) who coordinate patient flow, management of findings, and communication with the referring provider; a nurse navigator is a highly desirable part of the team, providing a central role in coordination and communications. Programs need to adhere to the CMS standards for the radiology infrastructure involved in LDCT screening, including equipment, interpretation, and reporting data to national registries such as the American College of Radiology (ACR) Lung Cancer Screening registry. ACR accredited imaging facilities for lung cancer screening may be found at https://www.acraccreditation.org/accredited-facility-search.

Bernstein and colleagues[52] and other investigators[42,43] point out that integration of data regarding lung cancer screening into the EMR continues to be problematic, because information that helps identify patients who are appropriate candidates for screening is not easy to enter. The pack-year smoking history, for example, often is recorded in a free text box. Referring physicians should be able to use EMRs as a tool to prompt screening discussions with eligible patients, find tools for SDM discussions, and refer patients to screening centers. Referring clinicians may have EMR systems that differ from those at screening centers, complicating referral as well as efforts at the nodule management clinic of identification, screening/results management, communication, and follow-up for repeat annual LDCT. EMRs also need to be structured in such a way that both referring providers and screening centers are not hampered by the required documentation for screening to justify the procedure and obtain reimbursement. Fathi and colleagues[53] discuss the benefits and challenges of using the EMR to support lung cancer screening, including the key elements of EMR software systems needed for this task. They point out that EMRs should support the referral process, patient data, tracking and navigation, and communication within the screening/nodule management center and with referring clinicians.

A standardized report for communication with referring providers, nodule management, and data reporting should be used, as discussed by the ACCP[51] or the ACR Lung Imaging Reporting and Data System (Lung-RADS) system.[54] Use of standardized reporting protocols with coordination by the nurse navigator allows for better nodule management and follow-up, including incidental findings.

SUMMARY

Lung cancer screening with LDCT provides an opportunity to save lives by early detection of the deadliest cancer in the United States. Uptake of lung cancer screening has been quite low, but anecdotal reports and a survey of 10 states suggest improvement. Clinician and patient education, integration of lung cancer screening protocols into EMR, support for SDM and tobacco cessation, and improved communication between referral centers and providing clinicians are all important areas for improvement for lung cancer screening to reach its potential in reducing morbidity and mortality from lung cancer.

DISCLOSURE

Dr T. Houston has no financial or other conflicts of interest to disclose.

REFERENCES

1. Miser WF. Cancer screening in the primary care setting: the role of the primary care physician in screening for breast, cervical, colorectal, lung, ovarian, and prostate cancers. Prim Care 2007;34(1):137–67.
2. Siegel RL, Miller KD, Ahmedin J. Cancer statistics, 2020. CA Cancer J Clin 2020; 70(1):7–30.
3. Cronin KA, Lake AJ, Scott S, et al. Annual report to the nation on the status of cancer, part I: national cancer statistics. Cancer 2018;124(13):2785–800.
4. Midthun DE. Screening for lung cancer. Clin Chest Med 2011;32:659–68.
5. Fontana RS. The Mayo lung project: a perspective. Cancer 2000;89(11 Suppl): 2352–5.
6. Eddy D. ACS report on the cancer-related health checkup. CA Cancer J Clin 1980;30:193–240.
7. American Academy of Family Physicians. New guidelines for cancer detection create stir. Am Fam Physician 1980;21(5):203–4.
8. American Cancer Society. Survey of physicians' attitudes and practices in early cancer detection. CA Cancer J Clin 1985;35(4):197–213.
9. McPhee SJ, Bird JA. Implementation of cancer prevention guidelines in clinical practice. J Gen Intern Med 1990;5(5 Suppl):S116–22.
10. Oken MM, Hocking WC, Kvale PA, et al. Screening by chest radiograph and lung cancer mortality. The Prostate, Lung, Colorectal, and Ovarian (PLCO) randomized trial. JAMA 2011;306(17):1865–73.
11. Kaneko M, Kusumoto M, Kobayashi T, et al. Computed tomography screening for lung carcinoma in Japan. Cancer 2000;89:2485–8.
12. Henschke CI. Early lung cancer action project: overall design and findings from baseline screening. Cancer 2000;89:2474–82.
13. Diederich S, Wormanns D, Lenzen H, et al. Screening for asymptomatic early bronchogenic carcinoma with low dose CT of the chest. Cancer 2000;89:2483–4.

14. van Klaveren RJ, Habbema JDF, Pedersen JH, et al. Lung cancer screening by low-dose spiral computed tomography. Eur Respir J 2001;18:857–66.

15. Pedersen JH, Dirksen A, Olsen JH. [Screening for lung cancer with low-dosage CT]. Ugeskr Laeger 2002;164:167–70.

16. Henschke CI, McCauley DI, Yankelevitz DF, et al. Early Lung Cancer Action Project: overall design and findings from baseline screening. Lancet 1999;354: 99–105.

17. Swensen SJ, Jett JR, Hartman TE, et al. CT screening for lung cancer: five-year prospective experience. Radiology 2005;235:259–65.

18. Diederich S, Wormanns D, Semik M, et al. Screening for early lung cancer with low-dose spiral CT: prevalence in 817 asymptomatic smokers. Radiology 2002; 222:773–81.

19. Pastorino U, Bellomi M, Landoni C, et al. Early lung cancer detection with spiral CT and positron emission tomography in heavy smokers: two-year results. Lancet 2003;362:593–7.

20. Sobue T, Moriyama N, Kaneko M, et al. Screening for lung cancer with low-dose helical computed tomography: anti-lung cancer association project. J Clin Oncol 2002;20:911–20.

21. Henschke CI, Naidich DP, Yankelevitz DF, et al. Early Lung Cancer Action Project: initial findings on repeat scanning. Cancer 2001;92:153–9.

22. The International Early Lung Cancer Action Program Investigators. Survival of patients with stage I lung cancer detected on CT screening. N Engl J Med 2006;355: 1763–71.

23. Aberle D, Adams A, Berg C. Reduced lung-cancer mortality with low-dose computed tomographic screening. N Engl J Med 2011;365(5):395–409.

24. Wood DE, Eapen GA, Ettinger DS, et al. Lung cancer screening. J Natl Compr Canc Netw 2012;10(2):240–65.

25. Wender R, Fontham ET, Barrera E Jr, et al. American Cancer Society lung cancer screening guidelines. CA Cancer J Clin 2013;63:107–17.

26. Moyer VA, U.S. Preventive Services Task Force. Screening for lung cancer: U.S. Preventive Services Task Force recommendation statement. Ann Intern Med 2014;160(5):330–8.

27. Compilation of Patient Protection and Affordable Care Act. Washington, DC: Senate and House of Representatives of the United States of America, 2010. Available at: http://housedocs.house.gov/energycommerce/ppacacon.pdf. Accessed, July 1, 2020.

28. American Academy of Family Physicians. Clinical recommendations. Lung cancer. Available at: https://www.aafp.org/patient-care/clinical-recommendations/all/lung-cancer.html. Accessed April 8, 2020.

29. United States Centers for Medicare and Medicaid Services. Decision Memo for Screening for Lung Cancer with Low Dose Computed Tomography (LDCT) (CAG-00439N). 2014. Available at: cms.gov/medicare-coverage-database/details/ncadecision-memo.aspx?NCAId5274. Accessed October 15, 2014.

30. de Koning HJ, van der Aalst CM, de Jong PA, et al. Reduced lung-cancer mortality with volume CT screening in a randomized trial. N Engl J Med 2020; 382(6):503–13.

31. Dawson Q. NELSON trial: reduced lung cancer mortality with volume CT scanning. Lancet Respir Med 2020;8:236.

32. Duffy SW, Field JK. Mortality reduction with low dose CT screening for lung cancer. N Engl J Med 2020;382(6):572–3.

33. Richards TB, Doria-Rose VP, Ashwini S, et al. Lung cancer screening inappropriate with U.S. Preventive Services Task Force recommendations. Am J Prev Med 2019;56(1):66–73.
34. Lewis JA, Chen H, Weaver KE, et al. Low provider knowledge Is associated with Less evidence-based lung cancer screening. J Natl Compr Canc Netw 2019; 17(4):339–46.
35. Klabunde CN, Marcus PM, Han PK, et al. Lung cancer screening practices of primary care physicians: results from a national survey. Ann Fam Med 2012;10(2): 102–10.
36. Hoffman RM, Sussman AL, Getrich CM, et al. Attitudes and beliefs of primary care providers in New Mexico about lung cancer screening using low-dose computed tomography. Prev Chronic Dis 2015;12:E108.
37. Ersek JL, Eberth JM, McDonnell KK, et al. Knowledge of, attitudes toward, and use of low-dose computed tomography for lung cancer screening among family physicians. Cancer 2016;122(15):2324–31.
38. Eberth JM, McDonnell KK, Sercy E, et al. A national survey of primary care physicians: Perceptions and practices of low-dose CT lung cancer screening. Prev Med Rep 2018;11:93–9.
39. Rajupet S, Doshi D, Wisnivesky JP, et al. Attitudes about lung cancer screening: primary care providers versus specialists. Clin Lung Cancer 2017;(6):e417–23.
40. Richards TB, Soman A, Thomas CC, et al. Screening for lung cancer - 10 states, 2017. MMWR Morb Mortal Wkly Rep 2020;69(8):201–6.
41. Jemal A, Fedewa SA. Lung cancer screening with low-dose computed tomography in the United States-2010 to 2015. JAMA Oncol 2017;3:1278–81.
42. Pham D, Bhandari S, Pinkston C, et al. Lung cancer screening registry reveals low-dose CT screening remains heavily underutilized. Clin Lung Cancer 2020; 21:e206–11.
43. Coughlin JM, Zang Y, Terranella S, et al. Understanding barriers to lung cancer screening in primary care. J Thorac Dis 2020;12(5):2536–44.
44. Melzer AC, Golden SE, Ono SS, et al. We just never have enough time": Clinician views of lung cancer screening processes and implementation. Ann Am Thorac Soc 2020. https://doi.org/10.1513/AnnalsATS.202003-262OC.
45. U.S. Department of Health and Human Services. Smoking cessation: a report of the surgeon general. Atlanta (GA): U.S. Department of Health and Human Services, Centers for Disease Control and Prevention, National Center for Chronic Disease Prevention and Health Promotion, Office on Smoking and Health; 2020.
46. Kathuria H, Koppelman E, Borrelli B, et al. Patient-physician discussions on lung cancer screening: a missed teachable moment to promote smoking cessation. Nicotine Tob Res 2020;22(3):431–9.
47. Fucito LM, Czabafy S, Hendricks PS, et al. Pairing smoking-cessation services with lung cancer screening: A clinical guideline from the Association for the Treatment of Tobacco Use and Dependence and the Society for Research on Nicotine and Tobacco. Cancer 2016;122(8):1150–9.
48. Tanner NT, Silvestri GA. Shared decision-making and lung cancer screening: let's get the conversation started. Chest 2019;155(1):21–4.
49. Hill PA. Current state of shared decision-making for CT lung cancer screening and improvement strategies. J Patient Exp 2020;7(1):49–52.
50. Lowenstein LM, Deyter GMR, Nishi S, et al. Shared decision-making conversations and smoking cessation interventions: critical components of low-dose CT lung cancer screening programs. Transl Lung Cancer Res 2018;7(3):254–71.

51. Mazzone P, Powell CA, Arenberg D, et al. Components necessary for high-quality lung cancer screening: American College of Chest Physicians and American Thoracic Society Policy Statement. Chest 2015;147:295–303.

52. Bernstein MA, Ronk M, Ebright MI. Establishing a lung cancer screening program in a non-university hospital. AME Med J 2018;3:102.

53. Fathi JT, White CS, Greenberg GM, et al. The integral role of the electronic health record and tracking software in the implementation of lung cancer screening-a call to action to developers: a white paper from the National Lung Cancer Round-table. Chest 2019. https://doi.org/10.1016/j.chest.2019.12.004 [pii:S0012-3692(19)34453-34458].

54. American College of Radiology. Lung CT screening, reporting and data system (Lung RADS). 2019. Available at: https://www.acr.org/Clinical-Resources/Reporting-and-Data-Systems/Lung-Rads. Accessed April 8, 2020.

Screening for Prostate Cancer

Sigrid V. Carlsson, MD, PhD, MPH[a,b,c], Andrew J. Vickers, PhD[d,*]

KEYWORDS

- Prostate cancer • Screening • Prostate-specific antigen • Biomarkers
- Magnetic resonance imaging

KEY POINTS

- Prostate-specific antigen (PSA) screening can reduce the risk of metastatic prostate cancer and death from the disease but is also associated with major harms, including overdiagnosis and overtreatment, with concomitant urinary, sexual, and bowel dysfunction.
- Primary care physicians can follow 7 simple steps that will dramatically reduce the harms of PSA screening while preserving its benefits.
- Patients need to be informed of the need for conservative management of low-grade prostate cancer and referred to urologists who promote active surveillance.
- Primary care physicians need to develop relationships with urologists who advocate conservative approaches to biopsy and treatment.

INTRODUCTION
Epidemiology

Prostate cancer is a major public health problem across the globe. With 1.3 million new cases and 359,000 deaths in 2018, prostate cancer is the second most common cancer and the fifth leading cause of cancer death in men worldwide. It is the commonest cancer in men in more than half of the countries of the world (105 of 185) and the leading cause of cancer death in men in 46 countries. The highest rates are seen in the Caribbean. Prostate cancer mortality has been decreasing

Funding: S.V. Carlsson's and A.J. Vickers's work was supported in part by funding from National Institutes of Health/National Cancer Institute (P30 CA008748, P50 CA92629, U01 CA199338-02), the Prevent Cancer Foundation, and Sidney Kimmel Center for Prostate and Urologic Cancers. S.V. Carlsson is also funded by a National Institutes of Health/National Cancer Institute Transition Career Development Award (K22 CA234400).
[a] Department of Surgery (Urology Service), Memorial Sloan Kettering Cancer Center, New York, NY, USA; [b] Department of Epidemiology and Biostatistics, Memorial Sloan Kettering Cancer Center, New York, NY, USA; [c] Department of Urology, Institute of Clinical Sciences, Sahlgrenska Academy at University of Gothenburg, Gothenburg, Sweden; [d] Department of Epidemiology and Biostatistics, Memorial Sloan Kettering Cancer Center, 485 Lexington Avenue, New York, NY 10065, USA
* Corresponding author.
E-mail address: vickersa@mskcc.org

in many countries because of screening, early detection, and improved treatment (eg, Northern America, Northern and Western Europe, Oceania, and developed countries of Asia) but increasing in several countries (eg, Central and South America, Central and Eastern European countries, many countries in Asia) possibly because of changes in risk factors, a more Westernized lifestyle, and limited access to treatment.[1]

Current Evidence for Prostate Cancer Screening

Localized prostate cancer is asymptomatic. By the time symptoms become present, the disease is generally too advanced for cure. Indeed, one of the most common presentations of prostate cancer before the advent of screening was paralysis, related to spinal cord metastasis. Therefore, the concept of screening is particularly appealing for prostate cancer, because it provides an opportunity to identify the disease at a curable stage. Research into a test that could detect prostate cancer earlier led to the discoveries of the blood test prostate-specific antigen (PSA), first isolated and defined in the 1970s.[2–4] Several screening studies in the late1980s to early 1990s showed that the PSA test could identify more prostate cancers at an organ-confined, clinically localized stage as compared with evaluations for palpable tumors by digital rectal examination, which set the stage for a widespread adoption of PSA testing, particularly in the United States, resulting in a rapid surge in prostate cancer incidence.[5–10]

There is level 1 evidence for PSA screening from large-scale randomized controlled trials, comparing regular PSA screening of men aged 50 to 70 every 2 to 4 years with no invitation to screening. The European Randomized Study of Screening for Prostate Cancer (ERSPC) reports a reduction in prostate cancer mortality by 20% (rate ratio [RR] 0.80, 95% confidence interval [CI] 0.72–0.89, $P<.001$) at 16 years of follow-up in favor of screening.[11] At this follow-up, the number needed to invite to screening to prevent 1 prostate cancer death is reported to be 570, and the number needed to diagnose is 18. The corresponding estimates from the Swedish Göteborg-1 trial with 18 years of follow-up are a reduction in prostate cancer mortality of 35% (RR 0.65, 95% CI 0.49–0.87, $P = .003$). To prevent 1 death from prostate cancer at 18 years, the number needed to invite to screening was 231, and the number needed to diagnose was 10. In contrast, at 17 years of follow-up in the US Prostate, Lung, Colorectal and Ovarian (PLCO) Cancer Screening Trial, there was no significant difference in prostate cancer mortality between the screening arm compared with the usual care arm (RR 0.93, 95% CI 0.81–1.08, $P = .4$).[12] However, this has been attributed to a high degree of contamination of PSA testing in the usual care arm, with more than 50% of patients randomized to no screening nonetheless undergoing PSA testing.[13,14] Statistical models have been used to reconcile the differences in implementation and settings and have reported that both trials provide compatible evidence that screening reduces prostate cancer mortality: estimated at 25%–31% in ERSPC and 27%–32% in PLCO, respectively.[15] Similarly, there is well-documented evidence from large, prospective observational studies regarding the prognostic utility of measuring a man's baseline PSA level in midlife to determine subsequent risk of future life-threatening prostate cancer.[16–21]

The age-specific prostate cancer mortality in the United States is decreased by 50% from peak rates because of PSA screening and improvements in treatment, but recently, this trend has been flattening because of recommendations against PSA screening in previous years, mainly the 2012 US Preventive Services Task Force guideline.[10,22] Studies now document a recent increase in metastatic prostate cancer.[23–26]

Controversies

PSA screening can have several beneficial effects. Most men have a "normal" PSA value less than the cutoff for further evaluation, and up to 97% of men report some reassurance with PSA screening.[27] Screening can reduce a man's risk of developing metastatic prostate cancer and dying from the disease.[11,28] For every prevented death from prostate cancer, a life is lengthened by 8 years on average.[29]

However, screening can also induce many undesired effects, including anxiety from false positive PSA tests and complications from further investigation with prostate biopsy, including hospitalization for infectious complications or rectal bleeding.[30] One major harm of PSA screening is overdiagnosis, that is, the diagnosis of indolent, slow-growing prostate cancer that would otherwise not be diagnosed during the man's lifetime.[31–33] Indolent disease is typically defined in terms of cancer grade. Gleason score 6, also termed grade group 1, is low-grade cancer that does not require immediate treatment.[34] High-grade disease, for which treatment should be considered, is defined as Gleason score 7 (grade group 2) or higher. Overdiagnosis turns healthy men into patients, which may take its toll on psychological well-being and quality of life.[35,36] Most importantly, over the past 2 decades, most men with low-risk prostate cancer in the United States underwent treatment with surgery and radiation. Such overtreatment has no, or almost no, benefit in terms of mortality reduction but leads to important and persistent side effects, most notably, urinary and erectile dysfunction.[37] In recent years, there has been a large shift in the treatment trends with more than half of men with low-risk disease now being recommended what is called active surveillance as the first management option, that is, careful monitoring with repeated testing and examinations and a switch to curative treatment upon signs of disease progression.[38–40] Avoiding overtreatment of indolent prostate cancer is crucial because active treatment with surgery, radiation, or ablative focal therapies can have significant impact on men's quality of life. Many years after treatment with radical prostatectomy or radiotherapy for favorable-risk prostate cancer, significant deterioration still persists in a substantial proportion of men in one or many functional domains: sexual function, urinary function (incontinence), and bowel function.[37,41] Modeling the lifetime effects of annual PSA screening between ages 55 and 69 versus no screening, Heijnsdijk and colleagues[29] estimated a loss of 23% of life-years gained with screening, primarily because of impaired quality of life owing to long-term side effects from treatment.

Current Guidelines

Table 1 gives a summary of examples of current PSA screening recommendations from major guideline groups in the United States and Europe. The guidelines are consistent in recommending shared decision making before starting screening and that the age range for screening should be around 45 to 70. There is some minor variation in the starting age (45–55) and the criteria for an upper age limit. The proposal for screening outlined in the clinical care points in later discussion is based on the Memorial Sloan Kettering Cancer Center recommendations[42] but are close to those of other groups.

CLINICAL CARE POINTS

In later discussion, the authors propose 7 steps for primary care doctors[42,43] (**Box 1**). The authors' proposal is based on the following principles. First, primary care is time-pressured, and primary care physicians cannot be expected to have in-depth subspecialty knowledge. Hence, the goal is to make shared decision making and the

Table 1
Examples of current guidelines for prostate cancer screening in 2020

Guideline Group	Reference, Year	Age to Start	Age to Stop
National Comprehensive Cancer Network (NCCN)	Carroll et al,[65] 2019	40–45	75 (continue in select cases)
Memorial Sloan Kettering Cancer Center (MSK)	Vickers et al,[42] 2016	45	60 for men with PSA <1 ng/mL, otherwise 70 (continue based on general health and prior PSAs)
European Association of Urology (EAU)– European Association of Nuclear Medicine (EANM)– European Society for Radiotherapy & Oncology (ESTRO)– European Society of Urogenital Radiology (ESUR)– International Society of Geriatric Oncology (SIOG)	Mottet et al,[40] 2020	50 45 if family history or African American 40 if carrying BRCA2 mutations	<15-y life expectancy (stop based on life expectancy and performance status)
American Urological Association (AUA)	Carter et al,[66] 2013[a]	55	70 (or <10–15 y life expectancy)
US Preventive Services Task Force (USPSTF)	Force USPST et al,[67] 2018	55 (shared decision making)	70 (recommends against)
American Cancer Society (ACS)	Wolf et al,[68] 2010	50 (shared decision making)	<10-y life expectancy

For additional examples of recommendations for PSA screening from various guideline groups, please see recent comprehensive reviews.
[a] Published 2013; Reviewed and validity confirmed 2018.
Data from Refs.[69,70]

subsequent screening algorithm relatively simple. Second, ensuring that PSA screening does more good than harm is primarily a matter of making sure that it does less harm: the recommendations reflect a "harm-reduction" approach. Third, given that there is great variability within urology with respect to compliance with clinical practice guidelines, the authors do make it incumbent upon primary care physicians to check that any urologists to whom they refer patients are engaging in best practices (described in points 5, 6, and 7).

1. **Get consent for prostate cancer screening, preferably using the "Simple Schema" decision aid.**

Box 1
Key practice points for primary care physicians

1. Get consent for prostate cancer screening, preferably using the "Simple Schema" decision aid.

2. PSA screening is only for healthy men aged 45 to 70.

3. Tailor screening frequency based on PSA level and cease screening for men older than 60 unless PSA is higher than median (1 ng/mL).

4. For men with elevated PSA (≥3 ng/mL), repeat PSA.

5. Use secondary tests, such as marker or imaging before biopsy, or only refer to urologists who do so.

6. Only refer to urologists who recommend active surveillance to almost all patients with low-grade cancer.

7. Preferably refer to urologists at major academic centers.

Prostate cancer screening is a preference-sensitive decision with important consequences. As such, it is important to obtain informed consent from patients following shared decision making. Although this only generally needs to occur once, informed consent is required to enter into a screening regimen, not for each and every PSA test, there are valid concerns as to the time required given the constraints of a busy primary care practice. Some guidelines recommend practices that are difficult to implement, such as one whereby patients are informed about 16 separate facts on PSA and are asked 12 questions about their preferences.[44] The authors developed what is known as the "Simple Schema"[45] (**Box 2**) for primary care physicians, which does not require knowledge above and beyond what any primary care physician would be expected to know, is brief, and focuses on harm reduction. The critical step is to warn patients about the risk that PSA screening will lead to the identification of low-risk disease and the need to avoid aggressive treatment in such cases. Early emphasis on active surveillance as the optimal management strategy for low-risk disease is critical.

A common question among primary care physicians is whether they should more strongly endorse PSA screening for men at higher risk, such as African Americans, or those with a family history or a genetic disposition. In brief, there is no reason to think that the benefit-to-harm ratio of PSA screening varies sufficiently for higher risk groups to mandate screening. Moreover, attempts to tailor PSA screening based on genomic risk, what are known as "polygenic risk scores," have not shown clinical utility for population-based screening.[46–49]

2. **PSA screening is only for healthy men aged 45 to 70.**

It is widely known that the introduction of PSA screening has led to widespread overdiagnosis. What is less widely recognized is that overdiagnosis is highly age dependent. Indeed, nearly half of the overdiagnosis associated with the introduction of PSA testing occurred in men aged older than 70.[50] Critically, PSA testing is of doubtful value in men aged older than 70: the hazard ratio for prostate cancer mortality for men older than 70 reported by the ERSPC is 1.18 (95% CI 0.81–1.72), that is, likely no benefit and, at most, about a 20% reduction in the risk of death from prostate cancer.[51] Hence, stopping

---

Box 2
Decision aid for primary care physicians for shared decision making about prostate cancer screening: the "Simple Schema"[45]

Key facts about prostate cancer and screening
- Prostate cancer is common: most men will develop it if they live long enough.
- Although only a small proportion of men with prostate cancer die of the disease, the best evidence shows that screening reduces the risk for prostate cancer death.
- Screening detects many low-risk or "indolent" cancer cases.
- In the United States, most low-risk cancer is treated, and the treatment itself can lead to complications, such as incontinence, erectile dysfunction, and bowel problems.

Key take-home messages
- The goal of screening is to find aggressive prostate cancer early and cure it before it spreads beyond the prostate.
- Most cancer cases found by screening do not need to be treated and can be safely managed by a program of careful monitoring known as "active surveillance."
- If you choose to be screened, there is a good chance that you will be diagnosed with low-risk cancer, and you may face pressure from your physicians or family to treat it.

Discrete decision
- If you are concerned that you would be uncomfortable knowing that you have cancer and not treating it, screening may not be for you.
- If you are confident that you would only accept treatment for aggressive cancer and would not be unduly worried about living with a diagnosis of low-risk disease, you are probably a good candidate for screening.

Reproduced with permission from Vickers AJ, Edwards K, Cooperberg MR, Mushlin AI. A simple schema for informed decision making about prostate cancer screening. Annals of Internal Medicine. 2014;161:441-442. https://www.acpjournals.org/doi/10.7326/M14-0151.

---

screening at 70 will have a large effect on overdiagnosis with little, if any, effect on mortality. Note that by ceasing screening, it is meant that PSA tests are generally discouraged in an asymptomatic man older than 70 with PSA levels in the normal range (ie, <3 ng/mL). Follow-up of older men older than 70 with PSA levels higher than 3 ng/mL is a matter of clinical judgment, taking into account the age and general health of the man (denoted "PSA surveillance").[52] Note also that it is reasonable to cease screening earlier than age 70 for men who have important comorbidities or to continue screening in a 70 year old in exceptional health.

As regards the starting age for screening, it has been shown at age 45, but not before, it is possible to identify a subgroup of men who are at important risk of prostate cancer morbidity or mortality within 10 years.[21] The yield is relatively low, that is, very few young men have an elevated PSA, and some commentators have therefore made the reasonable suggestion that screening start at 50 instead, based on this being the lowest age included in the ERSPC randomized trial. On the other hand, because younger men have a longer life-expectancy, they will lose a greater number of quality-adjusted life-years from cancer-related death and are at low risk for overdiagnosis. It has also been shown that, because PSA is a far stronger predictor of prostate cancer–specific mortality than race or family history, age at the start of screening should be the same for essentially all men.[53]

3. **Tailor screening frequency based on PSA level and cease screening for men older than 60 unless PSA is higher than median (1 ng/mL).**

PSA is not only diagnostic of the current risk of prostate cancer but highly prognostic of future risk.[16–21] Moreover, because prostate cancer is generally slow growing, screening intervals can safely be extended for men with low PSA. There are clear data that men with a low PSA are highly unlikely to develop aggressive prostate cancer within an 8- to 10-year period.[20,21,54] This finding has led to the "traffic light" algorithm as follows[42]:

- PSA less than 1 ng/mL: green light. Repeat PSA at a 8- to 10-year interval.
- PSA 1 to 2.99 ng/mL: amber light: Repeat PSA at a 2- to 4-year interval.
- PSA ≥3 ng/mL: red light. Consider further workup.

Fully 90% of prostate cancer deaths by age 85 occur in men with PSA above the median of 1 ng/mL at age 60.[20] It has also been shown that men with low PSA who continue to get screened are at some risk of overdiagnosis but receive no mortality benefit compared with if they had ceased screening.[17,54] Hence, men with PSA less than 1 ng/mL at age 60 should cease screening.

4. **For men with elevated PSA (≥3 ng/mL), repeat PSA.**

Many men will experience a temporary increase in PSA related to benign disease. For instance, in a landmark *JAMA* paper, 44% of men with PSA greater than 4 and 40% of those with PSA greater than 2.5 returned to normal PSA within 1 year.[55] A typical recommendation is that PSA should be repeated 4 to 6 weeks after an abnormal PSA.

5. **Use secondary tests, such as marker or imaging, before biopsy or only refer to urologists who do so.**

Only a small proportion of men with a moderately elevated PSA will have the sort of high-grade prostate cancer that is important to identify. Typically, for every 100 men with PSA greater than 3 ng/mL, approximately 70%, 20%, and 10%, respectively, will have benign disease, low-grade (indolent) prostate cancer, and high-grade cancer. There are now a wide variety of secondary tests that are available to determine which men with an elevated PSA should be subject to prostate biopsy. These secondary tests, which include biomarkers as shown in **Table 2**, as well as multiparametric MRI, have been shown to reduce both unnecessary biopsies and overdiagnosis of indolent disease.[56–58]

Some of these tests can be implemented in the primary care setting. For example, BioReference Laboratories offers a combined test for PSA, that is, when a PSA test is selected, the blood sample is automatically checked for the 4Kscore if PSA is elevated. However, in most cases, secondary tests, particularly MRI, are ordered by the urologist As such, it is incumbent on the primary care physician to develop a relationship with a urologist who takes a conservative approach to biopsy, incorporating secondary tests and only conducting biopsy on men shown to be at elevated risk of high-grade prostate cancer.

6. **Only refer to urologists who recommend active surveillance to almost all patients with low-grade cancer.**

The major harm of PSA screening is overtreatment, with consequent urinary, sexual, and bowel dysfunction.[37] Guidelines suggest that treatment should be restricted to men with high-grade disease. Men with Gleason score 6 (grade group 1) cancer should be managed conservatively, with an approach known as active surveillance, which involves PSA monitoring, repeat biopsies at regular intervals, and delayed intervention for men who progress to grade group 2 or higher disease. However, rates of active surveillance vary enormously between different practices: in 1 study, the proportion of low-risk men placed on active surveillance ranged from 25% to 80%.[59] As a result, the urologist

Table 2
Reflex biomarkers recommended by the National Comprehensive Cancer Network Guidelines v.2.2019 Prostate Cancer Early Detection

Initial Biopsy	Repeat Biopsy
% free PSA	% free PSA
Prostate Health Index (PHI)	Prostate Health Index (PHI)
4Kscore	4Kscore
ExoDx Prostate (IntelliScore)	ExoDx Prostate (IntelliScore)
	PCA3
	ConfirmMDx

Additional biomarkers (investigational): Michigan Prostate Score (MiPS), SelectMDx.
From Carroll P, Kellogg Parsons J, Andriole G, et al. NCCN Clinical Practice Guidelines in Oncology (NCCN Guidelines). Prostate Cancer Early Detection. V.2.2019. Available at: https://www.nccn.org/professionals/physician_gls/pdf/prostate_detection.pdf. 2019. With permission.

chosen by the primary care physician must take not only a conservative approach to biopsy but also a conservative approach to treatment. The primary care physician needs to ensure that the urologist raises active surveillance before biopsy and advises active surveillance to all, or nearly all, men with Gleason score 6 (grade group 1) disease.

7. **Preferably refer to urologists at major academic centers.**

The volume-outcome relationship is one of the most widely replicated findings in cancer medicine. In brief, both the chance of cure and the chance of side effects are strongly correlated with provider volume.[60–63] In 1 study, the risk of recurrence after prostate cancer was approximately half as great for surgeons with 250 radical prostatectomies compared with those who only had experience of 10 prior cases.[64] As such, primary care physicians should recommend to patients who require treatment for their prostate cancer, patients with grade group 2 or higher disease should be treated at a high-volume center. The easiest way to ensure this is to refer patients to a hospital that is designated by the National Cancer Institute as a Comprehensive Cancer Center (https://www.cancer.gov/research/nci-role/cancer-centers).

SUMMARY

PSA screening can importantly reduce the risk of death from prostate cancer but is also associated with major harms, overdiagnosis, and overtreatment, with attendant urinary, sexual, and bowel dysfunction. Following a few simple steps can dramatically reduce the risk of harm from PSA screening without materially reducing its benefits. In particular, patients need to be informed repeatedly of the need for conservative management of low-grade prostate cancer and referred to urologists who promote active surveillance. Primary care physicians need to develop relationships with urologists who advocate conservative approaches to biopsy and treatment.

DISCLOSURE

A.J. Vickers is named on a patent for a statistical method to detect prostate cancer. The patent application for the statistical model has been licensed and commercialized as the 4Kscore by OPKO Diagnostics. A.J. Vickers receives royalties from sales of this test and owns stock options in OPKO.

REFERENCES

1. Bray F, Ferlay J, Soerjomataram I, et al. Global cancer statistics 2018: GLOBO-CAN estimates of incidence and mortality worldwide for 36 cancers in 185 countries. CA Cancer J Clin 2018;68(6):394–424.
2. Wang MC, Valenzuela LA, Murphy GP, et al. Purification of a human prostate specific antigen. Invest Urol 1979;17(2):159–63.
3. Hara M, Koyanagi Y, Inoue T, et al. [Some physico-chemical characteristics of " -seminoprotein", an antigenic component specific for human seminal plasma. Forensic immunological study of body fluids and secretion. VII]. Nihon Hoigaku Zasshi 1971;25(4):322–4.
4. Li TS, Beling CG. Isolation and characterization of two specific antigens of human seminal plasma. Fertil Steril 1973;24(2):134–44.
5. Stamey TA, Yang N, Hay AR, et al. Prostate-specific antigen as a serum marker for adenocarcinoma of the prostate. N Engl J Med 1987;317(15):909–16.
6. Catalona WJ, Smith DS, Ratliff TL, et al. Measurement of prostate-specific antigen in serum as a screening test for prostate cancer. N Engl J Med 1991;324(17): 1156–61.
7. Wang TY, Kawaguchi TP. Preliminary evaluation of measurement of serum prostate-specific antigen level in detection of prostate cancer. Ann Clin Lab Sci 1986;16(6):461–6.
8. Cooner WH, Mosley BR, Rutherford CL Jr, et al. Prostate cancer detection in a clinical urological practice by ultrasonography, digital rectal examination and prostate specific antigen. J Urol 1990;143(6):1146–52 [discussion: 1152–4].
9. Brawer MK, Chetner MP, Beatie J, et al. Screening for prostatic carcinoma with prostate specific antigen. J Urol 1992;147(3 Pt 2):841–5.
10. Siegel RL, Miller KD, Jemal A. Cancer statistics, 2019. CA Cancer J Clin 2019; 69(1):7–34.
11. Hugosson J, Roobol MJ, Mansson M, et al. A 16-yr follow-up of the European Randomized Study of screening for prostate cancer. Eur Urol 2019;76(1):43–51.
12. Pinsky PF, Miller E, Prorok P, et al. Extended follow-up for prostate cancer incidence and mortality among participants in the Prostate, Lung, Colorectal and Ovarian Randomized Cancer Screening Trial. BJU Int 2018;123(5):854–60.
13. Shoag JE, Mittal S, Hu JC. Reevaluating PSA testing rates in the PLCO Trial. N Engl J Med 2016;374(18):1795–6.
14. Pinsky PF, Blacka A, Kramer BS, et al. Assessing contamination and compliance in the prostate component of the Prostate, Lung, Colorectal, and Ovarian (PLCO) Cancer Screening Trial. Clin Trials 2010;7(4):303–11.
15. Tsodikov A, Gulati R, Heijnsdijk EAM, et al. Reconciling the effects of screening on prostate cancer mortality in the ERSPC and PLCO trials. Ann Intern Med 2017;167(7):449–55.
16. Vertosick EA, Haggstrom C, Sjoberg DD, et al. Prespecified four kallikrein marker model (4Kscore) at age 50 or 60 for early detection of lethal prostate cancer in a large population-based cohort of asymptomatic men followed for 20 years. J Urol 2020;204(2):281–8.
17. Kovac E, Carlsson SV, Lilja H, et al. Association of baseline prostate-specific antigen level with long-term diagnosis of clinically significant prostate cancer among patients aged 55 to 60 years: a secondary analysis of a cohort in the Prostate, Lung, Colorectal, and Ovarian (PLCO) Cancer Screening Trial. JAMA Netw Open 2020;3(1):e1919284.

18. Preston MA, Gerke T, Carlsson SV, et al. Baseline prostate-specific antigen level in midlife and aggressive prostate cancer in black men. Eur Urol 2019;75(3): 399–407.

19. Preston MA, Batista JL, Wilson KM, et al. Baseline prostate-specific antigen levels in midlife predict lethal prostate cancer. J Clin Oncol 2016;34(23):2705–11.

20. Vickers AJ, Cronin AM, Bjork T, et al. Prostate specific antigen concentration at age 60 and death or metastasis from prostate cancer: case-control study. BMJ 2010;341:c4521.

21. Vickers AJ, Ulmert D, Sjoberg DD, et al. Strategy for detection of prostate cancer based on relation between prostate specific antigen at age 40-55 and long term risk of metastasis: case-control study. BMJ 2013;346:f2023.

22. Moyer VA. Screening for prostate cancer: U.S. Preventive Services Task Force recommendation statement. Ann Intern Med 2012;157(2):120–34.

23. Fleshner K, Carlsson SV, Roobol MJ. The effect of the USPSTF PSA screening recommendation on prostate cancer incidence patterns in the USA. Nat Rev Urol 2017;14(1):26–37.

24. Kelly SP, Anderson WF, Rosenberg PS, et al. Past, current, and future incidence rates and burden of metastatic prostate cancer in the United States. Eur Urol Focus 2018;4(1):121–7.

25. Dalela D, Sun M, Diaz M, et al. Contemporary trends in the incidence of metastatic prostate cancer among US men: results from nationwide analyses. Eur Urol Focus 2019;5(1):77–80.

26. Bandini M, Mazzone E, Preisser F, et al. Increase in the annual rate of newly diagnosed metastatic prostate cancer: a contemporary analysis of the Surveillance, Epidemiology and End Results database. Eur Urol Oncol 2018;1(4):314–20.

27. Cantor SB, Volk RJ, Cass AR, et al. Psychological benefits of prostate cancer screening: the role of reassurance. Health Expect 2002;5(2):104–13.

28. Buzzoni C, Auvinen A, Roobol MJ, et al. Metastatic prostate cancer incidence and prostate-specific antigen testing: new insights from the European Randomized Study of screening for prostate cancer. Eur Urol 2015;68(5):885–90.

29. Heijnsdijk EA, Wever EM, Auvinen A, et al. Quality-of-life effects of prostate-specific antigen screening. N Engl J Med 2012;367(7):595–605.

30. Loeb S, Vellekoop A, Ahmed HU, et al. Systematic review of complications of prostate biopsy. Eur Urol 2013;64(6):876–92.

31. Loeb S, Bjurlin MA, Nicholson J, et al. Overdiagnosis and overtreatment of prostate cancer. Eur Urol 2014;65(6):1046–55.

32. Draisma G, Etzioni R, Tsodikov A, et al. Lead time and overdiagnosis in prostate-specific antigen screening: importance of methods and context. J Natl Cancer Inst 2009;101(6):374–83.

33. Welch HG, Kramer BS, Black WC. Epidemiologic signatures in cancer. N Engl J Med 2019;381(14):1378–86.

34. Klotz L. Active surveillance for low-risk prostate cancer. Curr Opin Urol 2017; 27(3):225–30.

35. Bellardita L, Villa S, Valdagni R. Living with untreated prostate cancer: predictors of quality of life. Curr Opin Urol 2014;24(3):311–7.

36. McIntosh M, Opozda MJ, Evans H, et al. A systematic review of the unmet supportive care needs of men on active surveillance for prostate cancer. Psychoncology 2019;28(12):2307–22.

37. Hoffman KE, Penson DF, Zhao Z, et al. Patient-reported outcomes through 5 years for active surveillance, surgery, brachytherapy, or external beam radiation

with or without androgen deprivation therapy for localized prostate cancer. JAMA 2020;323(2):149–63.

38. Cooperberg MR, Carroll PR. Trends in management for patients with localized prostate cancer, 1990-2013. JAMA 2015;314(1):80–2.

39. Loeb S, Byrne NK, Wang B, et al. Exploring variation in the use of conservative management for low-risk prostate cancer in the veterans affairs healthcare system. Eur Urol 2020;77(6):683–6.

40. Mottet N, Cornford P, van den Bergh R, et al. EAU-EANM-ESTRO-ESUR-SIOG Guidelines on Prostate Cancer 2020. Available at: https://uroweb.org/guideline/prostate-cancer/. Accessed September 2, 2020.

41. Johansson E, Steineck G, Holmberg L, et al. Long-term quality-of-life outcomes after radical prostatectomy or watchful waiting: the Scandinavian Prostate Cancer Group-4 randomised trial. Lancet Oncol 2011;12(9):891–9.

42. Vickers AJ, Eastham JA, Scardino PT, et al. The Memorial Sloan Kettering Cancer Center recommendations for prostate cancer screening. Urology 2016;91:12–8.

43. Vickers A, Carlsson S, Laudone V, et al. It ain't what you do, it's the way you do it: five golden rules for transforming prostate-specific antigen screening. Eur Urol 2014;66(2):188–90.

44. Feng B, Srinivasan M, Hoffman JR, et al. Physician communication regarding prostate cancer screening: analysis of unannounced standardized patient visits. Ann Fam Med 2013;11(4):315–23.

45. Vickers AJ, Edwards K, Cooperberg MR, et al. A simple schema for informed decision making about prostate cancer screening. Ann Intern Med 2014;161(6): 441–2.

46. Schumacher FR, Al Olama AA, Berndt SI, et al. Association analyses of more than 140,000 men identify 63 new prostate cancer susceptibility loci. Nat Genet 2018; 50(7):928–36.

47. Aly M, Wiklund F, Xu J, et al. Polygenic risk score improves prostate cancer risk prediction: results from the Stockholm-1 cohort study. Eur Urol 2011;60(1):21–8.

48. Pashayan N, Duffy SW, Neal DE, et al. Implications of polygenic risk-stratified screening for prostate cancer on overdiagnosis. Genet Med 2015;17(10):789–95.

49. Li-Sheng Chen S, Ching-Yuan Fann J, Sipeky C, et al. Risk prediction of prostate cancer with single nucleotide polymorphisms and prostate specific antigen. J Urol 2019;201(3):486–95.

50. Vickers AJ, Sjoberg DD, Ulmert D, et al. Empirical estimates of prostate cancer overdiagnosis by age and prostate-specific antigen. BMC Med 2014;12:26.

51. Schroder FH, Hugosson J, Roobol MJ, et al. Prostate-cancer mortality at 11 years of follow-up. N Engl J Med 2012;366(11):981–90.

52. Carlsson SV, Eastham JA, Crawford ED, et al. PSA surveillance in the septuagenarian": a proposed new terminology for clinical follow-up to assess risk of prostate cancer in men aged 70 years and older. Eur Urol 2020;78(2):136–7.

53. Vertosick EA, Poon BY, Vickers AJ. Relative value of race, family history and prostate specific antigen as indications for early initiation of prostate cancer screening. J Urol 2014;192(3):724–8.

54. Carlsson S, Assel M, Sjoberg D, et al. Influence of blood prostate specific antigen levels at age 60 on benefits and harms of prostate cancer screening: population based cohort study. BMJ 2014;348:g2296.

55. Eastham JA, Riedel E, Scardino PT, et al. Variation of serum prostate-specific antigen levels: an evaluation of year-to-year fluctuations. JAMA 2003;289(20): 2695–700.

56. Kearns JT, Lin DW. Improving the specificity of PSA screening with serum and urine markers. Curr Urol Rep 2018;19(10):80.

57. Kasivisvanathan V, Rannikko AS, Borghi M, et al. MRI-targeted or standard biopsy for prostate-cancer diagnosis. N Engl J Med 2018;378(19):1767–77.

58. Drost FH, Osses D, Nieboer D, et al. Prostate magnetic resonance imaging, with or without magnetic resonance imaging-targeted biopsy, and systematic biopsy for detecting prostate cancer: a Cochrane systematic review and meta-analysis. Eur Urol 2020;77(1):78–94.

59. Loppenberg B, Friedlander DF, Krasnova A, et al. Variation in the use of active surveillance for low-risk prostate cancer. Cancer 2018;124(1):55–64.

60. Eastham JA. Do high-volume hospitals and surgeons provide better care in urologic oncology? Urol Oncol 2009;27(4):417–21.

61. Savage CJ, Vickers AJ. Low annual caseloads of United States surgeons conducting radical prostatectomy. J Urol 2009;182(6):2677–9.

62. Vickers AJ, Savage CJ, Hruza M, et al. The surgical learning curve for laparoscopic radical prostatectomy: a retrospective cohort study. Lancet Oncol 2009; 10(5):475–80.

63. Bravi CA, Tin A, Vertosick E, et al. The impact of experience on the risk of surgical margins and biochemical recurrence after robot-assisted radical prostatectomy: a learning curve study. J Urol 2019;202(1):108–13.

64. Vickers AJ, Bianco FJ, Serio AM, et al. The surgical learning curve for prostate cancer control after radical prostatectomy. J Natl Cancer Inst 2007;99(15): 1171–7.

65. Carroll P, Kellogg Parsons J, Andriole G, et al. NCCN clinical practice guidelines in Oncology (NCCN guidelines). Prostate cancer early detection. V.2.2019. Available at: https://www.nccn.org/professionals/physician_gls/pdf/prostate_detection.pdf. Accessed September 2, 2020.

66. Carter HB, Albertsen PC, Barry MJ, et al. Early detection of prostate cancer: AUA Guideline. J Urol 2013;190(2):419–26.

67. Force USPST, Grossman DC, Curry SJ, et al. Screening for prostate cancer: US Preventive Services Task Force Recommendation Statement. JAMA 2018; 319(18):1901–13.

68. Wolf AMD, Wender RC, Etzioni RB, et al. American Cancer Society guideline for the early detection of prostate cancer update 2010. CA Cancer J Clin 2010;60(2): 70–98.

69. Filella X, Albaladejo MD, Allue JA, et al. Prostate cancer screening: guidelines review and laboratory issues. Clin Chem Lab Med 2019;57(10):1474–87.

70. Kohestani K, Chilov M, Carlsson SV. Prostate cancer screening-when to start and how to screen? Transl Androl Urol 2018;7(1):34–45.

Screening for Cervical Cancer

Terresa J. Eun, AB[a,b], Rebecca B. Perkins, MD, MSc[a,b,*]

KEYWORDS

- Cervical cytology • PAP test • HPV test • Cervical cancer screening

KEY POINTS

- HPV vaccination in adolescence is critical to preventing cervical cancer in young adults; screening is the key to preventing cervical cancer in adult patients.
- Achieving and maintaining high rates of cervical cancer screening in the 25- to 65-year-old population is the key to cervical cancer prevention.
- HPV testing detects more disease and achieves higher rates of cancer prevention than Pap testing; it can also be performed less frequently with superior results.
- Ensuring adequate screening between ages 45 and 65 is critical to preventing cervical cancer after age 65.
- Reminder/recall/tracking systems are necessary to ensuring that testing occurs when needed for individuals undergoing routine screening and for those undergoing surveillance after abnormalities.

HUMAN PAPILLOMAVIRUS INFECTION CAUSES CERVICAL CANCER: EPIDEMIOLOGY AND BACKGROUND

Each year in the United States, nearly 13,000 women develop cervical cancer and 4000 die from the disease.[1] However, most cases can be prevented with vaccination and screening because it is now understand that oncogenic human papillomavirus (HPV) infections cause nearly all cervical cancers.[2] Approximately 14 evolutionarily related HPV genotypes have oncogenic potential,[3,4] with HPV 16 and 18 alone being responsible for nearly 70% of cervical cancers.[3–5]

HPV is the most common sexually transmitted infection, with nearly half of Americans infected.[6,7] HPV is commonly acquired shortly after sexual debut,[8] with a peak incidence between the ages of 15 and 25 years. An estimated 80% of HPV infections that go on to cause cancer are acquired before age 26.[9] Although most infections regress spontaneously within 1 to 2 years, the longer the infection persists in a

a Department of Sociology, Stanford University, 120, 450 Serra Mall Wallenberg, Stanford, CA 94305, USA; b Department of Obstetrics and Gynecology, Boston University School of Medicine, Boston Medical Center, 85 East Concord Street, 6th Floor, Boston, MA 02118, USA
* Corresponding author. 850 Harrison Avenue, Dowling Building, 4th Floor, Boston, MA 02118.
E-mail address: rbperkin@bu.edu

Med Clin N Am 104 (2020) 1063–1078
https://doi.org/10.1016/j.mcna.2020.08.006
0025-7125/20/© 2020 Elsevier Inc. All rights reserved.
medical.theclinics.com

detectable state, the higher the risk of cervical precancer or cancer.[10,11] Cervical cancer precursors, or precancer, are described histopathologically as moderate to severe dysplasia, histologic high-grade squamous intraepithelial lesion (HSIL), or cervical intraepithelial neoplasia grades 2 and 3 (CIN2 or CIN3). Typically, precancers are diagnosed approximately 5 to 10 years following the initial oncogenic infection, with peak prevalence between ages 25 and 35.[12] If left untreated, approximately 30% of high-grade precancers eventually become invasive cancers.[11] Cervical cancer rates begin to rise in the mid-30s, peaking at ages 35 to 45 years, and remain high into older ages.[13,14]

PRIMARY PREVENTION: HUMAN PAPILLOMAVIRUS VACCINATION
Vaccination of Adolescents Reduces Precancers and Cancers

Because the role of HPV in cervical cancer is understood, there is access to primary prevention (vaccination) and secondary prevention (screening). Extensive evidence supports the effectiveness of HPV vaccination in early adolescence for preventing vaccine-type HPV infections, precancerous lesions, and cervical cancer in young adults. If the currently available vaccines provide lifelong protection, cervical cancer rates could be reduced by 85% for those who receive vaccination before they are exposed to oncogenic HPV.[15] Studies indicate that HPV vaccination leads to reductions in rates of HPV infection and HPV-related diseases at each step along the carcinogenic pathway. First, vaccination before sexual debut reduces vaccine-type oncogenic HPV infections by more than 90% in vaccinated individuals; unvaccinated individuals begin to benefit from herd immunity when vaccination rates exceed 50%.[16–18] As vaccine programs were introduced, epidemiologic analyses demonstrated the near-disappearance of genital warts in vaccinated populations, with strong evidence for protection of nonvaccinated males when female vaccination rates were high.[19] The second piece of population-level evidence is the demonstration of decreasing rates of cervical precancers among vaccinated populations[20–22] and decreased incidence of cervical precancers in vaccinated compared with unvaccinated individuals.[23,24] The final and most important finding is the observed decline in HPV-related cancers. Reduction in HPV-related cancers was first observed in long-term follow-up studies of the original vaccine trial participants, starting an average of 7 years following vaccination.[25] More recently, invasive cancer rates have declined among the 15- to 24-year-old population in the United States from the prevaccine to the postvaccine era.[26]

Vaccination of Young Adults Has Limited Population-Level Benefit

In contrast to vaccination of adolescents, vaccination of young adults has not been associated with reductions in cervical precancer or cancer in most studies because of high rates of HPV infection. Although clinical trials indicated vaccine efficacy through age 26 among women without evidence of previous infection, when women with preexisting infections were included in the analysis, vaccine efficacy decreased with age, with a 50% reduction noted for those initiating vaccination older than age 21.[27] Because most HPV infections are acquired in early young adulthood, vaccine effectiveness at the population level is lower for this age group. Analysis of a large prepaid health plan in California (Kaiser Permanente) demonstrated a 50% reduction in cervical precancer for young women vaccinated before age 18 but no reduction for those vaccinated at ages 18 and older compared with those who were never vaccinated.[28] Similarly, population-level data in Sweden indicated that vaccine effectiveness against precancer decreased with age, declining from 64% for those vaccinated before age 17, to 25% for vaccination at ages 17 to 19, to no benefit for when vaccination occurred at ages 20 to 29.[29]

Vaccination of Adults Aged 27 to 45 Does Not Have Population-Level Benefits

The Advisory Committee on Immunization Practices voted in 2019 to allow HPV vaccination of adults ages 27 to 45. They did not recommend routine vaccination for this population, but instead allowed for shared decision-making with individual patients.[30] Review of 11 clinical trials of vaccination in midadult women demonstrated near-universal seroconversion, and reductions in combined end points, which included HPV infections, genital warts, and histopathologic changes of low grade (CIN1) or higher.[30] No benefits were noted when restricting analyses to precancer or cancer end points only. HPV vaccines seemed to be safe in midadults, and the committee voted 10 to 4 in favor of shared clinical decision-making. Because of the limited benefits, the guideline states: "Catch-up HPV vaccination is not recommended for all adults aged greater than 26 years. Instead, shared clinical decision-making regarding HPV vaccination is recommended for some adults aged 27 through 45 years who are not adequately vaccinated." Because vaccination did not significantly reduce precancers and cancers in this population, guidelines further emphasize that, regardless of vaccination status, "Cervical cancer screening guidelines and recommendations should be followed."[30] Updated American Cancer Society (ACS) guidelines do not endorse vaccination of adults ages 27 to 45.[31]

SECONDARY PREVENTION: CERVICAL CANCER SCREENING
Evidence Supporting Screening in Adults

Population-level, organized screening programs have reduced cervical cancer rates by 50% to 80%.[32,33] In settings with robust screening programs, most cancers develop among those who are new to care or rarely screened.[34,35] Unequal access to screening is a key reason for the dramatic disparities in cervical cancer incidence and mortality seen between low-resource and high-resource countries,[36] and also between socially advantaged and disadvantaged individuals in the United States.[33] Cervical cancer screening programs function by identifying asymptomatic women with precancerous lesions to allow for diagnosis and treatment before cancer develops. Screening tests must be sensitive, reproducible, and easily performed and managed by primary care clinicians. Cervical cytology (Pap testing) was the mainstay of screening for decades, but HPV testing has taken on an increasingly important role as understanding of the role of HPV infection in cervical cancer development has improved.[37,38]

WHAT TESTS ARE USED FOR SCREENING?

Without question, the best screening test is the one that is performed. Cervical cytology (Pap testing), HPV primary screening, and cotesting using HPV and cytology all reduce cervical cancer incidence and mortality if guidelines are followed. However, there are advantages and disadvantages to the different screening tests.

Cervical Cytology (Pap Testing)

Cervical cytology involves a clinician performing a speculum examination and collecting a sample of cervical cells, which are either smeared onto a slide (conventional cytology) or placed into a liquid medium (liquid-based cytology), and sent to a laboratory for analysis by a cytopathologist. Examination of the cells can reveal normal-appearing cells, low-grade abnormalities, or high-grade abnormalities. Low-grade abnormalities, defined as atypical squamous cells of undetermined significance (ASC-US) or low-grade squamous intraepithelial lesion (LSIL), generally indicate evidence of HPV infection but are not immediately suggestive of a precancerous lesion. High-grade abnormalities, defined as HSIL, atypical squamous cells suggestive of high-grade, and atypical glandular cells, are highly correlated with high-grade histologic findings, which require excisional treatment to prevent the development of invasive cancer. Cytology is a specific test; if a high-grade abnormality is found, the likelihood of precancer is high. However, it is not a sensitive test; 30% to 50% of precancers are missed with each screening round.[39,40] Because of the low sensitivity, frequently repeated cytology testing over decades is needed to prevent cancer.[41,42]

Human Papillomavirus Primary Screening

HPV primary screening involves collection of a cervical or vaginal sample to detect the presence of an oncogenic HPV infection. Currently, available HPV tests in the United States involve clinician-collected cervical samples obtained via a speculum examination. However, the ability to detect an oncogenic HPV infection is similar when using a self-collected vaginal swab or a clinician-collected sample, making self-sampling a possible option for the future. A meta-analysis of 56 studies found that HPV assays using polymerase chain reaction technology were as sensitive with self-samples as with clinician-collected samples, although assays based on signal amplification were less sensitive.[43] mRNA assays also seems to be less sensitive when obtained via self-collection compared with clinician collection.[44] Trials are currently underway to define the parameters for broader use of self-collected samples. One advantage to self-sampling is the potential to increase screening participation in populations that currently experience high cancer rates because of lack of screening, specifically those living in low-resource settings either in low-income countries[45] or in low-resource settings within high-income countries.[46]

HPV testing, whether clinician-collected or self-collected, is more sensitive than cytology. A single HPV test detects 90% of precancers and cancers.[47] Thus, the negative predictive value (reassurance) of HPV testing is far better than cytology and allows safe extension of screening intervals.[48,49] Testing using HPV assays at 5-year intervals results in a lower risk of cancer and precancer than cytology testing at 3-year intervals.[49] Sequential negative HPV tests provide extensive protection, yielding a risk for high-grade precancer of fewer than 1 case per 1000 patients screened.[50,51]

Another advantage of HPV testing is superior detection of adenocarcinoma and its precursors compared with cytology.[52] Cytologic specimens often appear normal even when adenocarcinoma and adenocarcinoma in situ (AIS) are present, with the consequence that cytology-based screening programs that effectively reduce rates of squamous cancers do not reduce rates of adenocarcinomas and AIS.[47,53,54] Because HPV testing leads to earlier detection of squamous and glandular precancers (CIN3/AIS), incorporating HPV testing into cervical cancer screening programs reduces cancer incidence within 5 years and mortality within 8 years compared with cytology screening alone.[41,55]

Although randomized trials of Pap and HPV testing consistently demonstrate that HPV testing identifies precancers earlier, the proportion of abnormal results is higher when screening with HPV tests compared with cytology alone: 10% and 6%, respectively.[56] However, recommendations for repeat testing in 1 year rather than immediate colposcopic referral for HPV-positive tests with normal cytology results lead to similar or only marginally higher rates of referral to colposcopy.[38] Adhering to recommended screening intervals is important when using HPV testing for screening, because repeating the test too soon is more likely to detect transient HPV infections than precancer. This can increase emotional distress and financial burden without decreasing cancer incidence and mortality, so adherence to recommended intervals is important for realizing the benefits of HPV screening.[57] Of note, some HPV tests may be used alone, whereas others may only be used with concurrent cytology (cotesting).

Cotesting

Cotesting involves taking a cervical cytology sample and HPV test during the same examination. Samples are collected by a clinician during a speculum examination. Depending on which tests are used, cytology and HPV tests may be collected separately or both tests may be performed from a single liquid-based cytology sample. Similar to HPV testing alone, cotesting detects greater than 90% of precancers and cancers with a single screen.[47] Serial negative screens confer increasing protection, with one study of 990,013 women finding no cervical cancers and few precancers after two negative cotests.[51] Screening with cotesting slightly increases the sensitivity for detecting high-grade cervical precancers (CIN3 and AIS) and invasive cervical cancers compared with HPV testing alone, detecting approximately five additional cancers per million women screened.[47,58,59] Abnormal cytologic findings with negative HPV tests may also occur in advanced cancers, often caused by an abundance of necrotic tissue in the sample that obscures HPV test results. However, most advanced cancers are detected because of symptoms and are thus not preventable via screening of asymptomatic populations. A disadvantage of screening with cytology in addition to HPV testing is the number of abnormal results without a substantial reduction in the cancer burden. Modeling studies indicate that 640 colposcopies would be performed per cancer prevented when using HPV testing alone, compared with almost 1000 colposcopies per prevented cancer using cotesting.[60] Modeling a population of 100,000 individuals screened over their lifetimes, cotesting would prevent five additional cervical cancers and two deaths compared with HPV testing, but with about 50% more false-positive results and colposcopies.[60]

Screening Test Summary

The goal of a screening test is to accurately separate individuals at high risk of disease from those at low risk of disease, and to minimize false-negative results. By these parameters, HPV testing is clearly superior to cytology testing alone as a screening test for cervical cancer, because it detects far more precancerous lesions per screen. Adding cytology to HPV testing alone (cotesting) slightly increases the number of cases detected, but at the cost of more false-positive results and more invasive procedures (colposcopy with biopsy).

WHO SHOULD BE SCREENED?

Although there some areas of disagreement, most cervical cancer screening guidelines agree on which individuals should and should not be screened for cervical cancer (**Table 1**).[37,38,61,62]

Individuals Who Should Be Screened

- All individuals with a cervix (women who have not undergone hysterectomy with removal of the cervix and trans-men) ages 25 to 65 regardless of sexual history or sexual orientation.

Table 1
Comparison of ACS 2020, USPSTF 2018, and ACOG 2016 screening guidelines

Guideline Author	American Cancer Society (ACS) 2020	US Preventive Services Task Force (USPSTF) 2018	American College of Obstetricians and Gynecologists 2016
Age to start screening	25	21	21
Age to end screening	65[a]	65[a]	65[a]
Screening test options	HPV primary screening preferred for all ages; co-testing and cytology (Pap test) acceptable during transition	Cytology (Pap test) ages 21–29; HPV primary screening, co-testing, and cytology all equally acceptable ages 30–65	Cytology (Pap test) ages 21–29; HPV primary screening, co-testing, and cytology all equally acceptable ages 30–65; HPV primary screening every 3 y for ages 25–65 can be considered
Testing interval	5 y	3 y for cytology (Pap test); 5 y for HPV primary screening and co-testing	3 y for cytology (Pap test); 5 y for co-testing; 3 y for HPV primary screening
Individuals who have undergone hysterectomy with removal of the cervix for benign indications	Do not screen	Do not screen	Do not screen
Exclusions from screening guidelines	Screening guidelines do not apply to individuals with a history of cervical cancer or pre-cancer, DES in utero exposure, or immunocompromised, including HIV infection, as more frequent testing is typically recommended.		

[a] Criteria to end screening: 3 consecutive negative cytologies (Pap tests) or 2 negative screening HPV or co-tests within the past 10 y, without abnormal results during that time, with the most recent within the past 5 y and no history of pre-cancer (defined as CIN2 or higher) within the past 25 y.

- Individuals who have undergone hysterectomy with removal of the cervix only if they had a diagnosis of precancer or cancer before hysterectomy.
- Individuals older than age 65 who do not meet exit criteria. To fulfill exit criteria, a patient must have medical record documentation of two consecutive negative HPV tests or cotests or three consecutive negative Pap tests between ages 55 and 65 years, with no abnormal screening within that time, and no history of precancer (CIN2, CIN3, or AIS) within the past 25 years.

Screening applies only to asymptomatic individuals. Cervical cytology (Pap testing) should be performed as part of the work-up of abnormal uterine bleeding even if the patient is not due for a "screening" test.

Individuals Who Should Not Be Screened

- Individuals aged less than 21 years
- Individuals who have undergone hysterectomy for benign indications
- Individuals older than age 65 who fulfilled exit criteria

Age Less Than 21

All guidelines agree that screening should not occur before age 21 (unless the individual is human immunodeficiency virus positive) because the rates of HPV infection and minor cellular abnormalities are high, leading to the potential for overtreatment of lesions never destined to go on to become cancer. HPV infection rates peak shortly after sexual debut.[63] Most HPV infections and low-grade cytologic abnormalities (ASC-US, LSIL) regress within 1 to 2 years in young women[64,65] and even many high-grade lesions regress over time without treatment.[66,67]

Ages 21 to 24

Screening is recommended starting at age 21 in the 2016 American College of Obstetricians and Gynecologists (ACOG) and 2018 US Preventive Services Task Force (USPSTF) guidelines, but it is recommended starting at age 25 in the 2020 ACS guidelines.[62] Between 2012 and 2018, initiating screening at age 21 was believed to represent the best balance of the benefits of screening and harms of overtreatment. However, as HPV vaccination rates rise, the balance is shifting toward initiating screening later. ACS cites three primary reasons for raising the screening initiation age to 25 years. First, individuals who received on-time HPV vaccination are aging into this cohort, leading to a decline in precancers and cancers that is independent of screening.[26,28] Because vaccination has reduced rates of HPV 16/18 infections,[17] most abnormal cytology results represent transient infections with less aggressive oncogenic HPV types, which can lead to invasive diagnostic tests (eg, colposcopy with biopsy) but are unlikely to cause cancer.[28] Second, many high-grade lesions diagnosed at ages less than 25 are destined to regress without treatment.[67,68] Deferring unnecessary treatment in young women is important because some data indicate that treatment may lead to future pregnancy complications,[69,70] although other studies do not show this association.[71] Finally, initiating treatment at age 25 allows HPV testing at 5-year intervals to be recommended for all individuals, simplifying guidelines for clinicians.

Ages 25 to 65

All guidelines agree that screening is beneficial for this age group because organized screening programs consistently lead to decreases in cancer incidence and mortality.[37,38,61]

Age Greater Than 65

Women older than age 65 represent 20% of cervical cancers and have excess mortality compared with younger women.[14,72] However, studies indicate that many individuals diagnosed with cancer older than age 65 did not fulfill exit criteria as defined previously.[73,74] In addition, the sensitivity of cytology and HPV screening tests seems to decrease in older women,[34] and colposcopy also becomes more difficult because more lesions are found inside the endocervical canal after menopause, which are less amenable to colposcopic detection.[75] Therefore, emphasis is placed on ensuring adequate screening between ages 45 and 65, rather than continuing screening later in life. Note that women with screening test abnormalities must continue to screen until exit criteria are met.[76]

Hysterectomy with Removal of the Cervix

Because individuals without a cervix are at extraordinarily low risk for cervical cancer, screening should be discontinued following hysterectomy with removal of the cervix when performed for benign indications.[77] Following treatment of high-grade cervical precancer, individuals remain at risk of recurrent disease at the vaginal cuff, and should undergo screening for 25 years following their treatment (which may be <25 years after hysterectomy if they were treated with an excisional procedure and then went on to have a hysterectomy for another indication later).[76]

HOW SHOULD INDIVIDUALS BE FOLLOWED AFTER ABNORMAL RESULTS?
Surveillance: Interplay of Management and Screening

A substantial minority of women do not qualify for routine screening intervals. Up to 20% of women report at least one prior abnormal screening result,[78] and a cross-sectional analysis of a population screened with cotesting demonstrated that approximately 10% of women had an abnormal result.[56] Surveillance at shorter intervals is now recommended for a minimum of 10 years (four consecutive negative tests) after most abnormalities, which means that in any given primary care population, 10% to 20% of patients may not qualify for routine screening.[76] The 2019 ASCCP Risk-Based Management Consensus Guidelines[76] recommend follow-up surveillance at 1 year for abnormalities with an immediate risk of precancer (CIN3+) less than 4%, but a 5-year risk greater than 0.55%. Results that fall into the 1-year surveillance category include low-grade results not requiring colposcopy (eg, normal cytology with a positive HPV test), follow-up after a colposcopy confirming low-grade abnormalities (CIN1), or during the initial period of intensive follow-up after treatment of a high-grade lesion (histologic HSIL or CIN2/CIN3).

Surveillance at 3 years is recommended for individuals whose cumulative 5-year CIN3+ risk falls between 0.015% and 0.054%.[76] Surveillance with HPV testing or cotesting at 3-year intervals is recommended for long-term surveillance following initial resolution of most abnormalities. At this time, even after three consecutive negative follow-up HPV tests or cotests, data indicate that risks remain in the range for which 3-year follow-up is recommended. With currently available data, return to routine screening is currently recommended for only two scenarios:

1. HPV-negative ASC-US followed by a negative HPV test or cotest, and

2. Minimally abnormal screening results (HPV-positive negative for intraepithelial lesion or malignancy [NILM], HPV-positive ASC-US, HPV-positive LSIL), with low-grade disease confirmed at colposcopy (biopsy of CIN1 or normal) followed by three consecutive negative HPV tests or cotests.

PRACTICAL IMPLICATIONS

Because routine screening intervals do not apply to up to 20% of individuals, risk-stratification and long-term tracking of primary care populations is crucial. When annual well-woman examinations were the standard of care, visits could easily be scheduled by office staff, and patients could easily remember when their next visit was due. With more nuanced approaches to cervical cancer screening and surveillance following abnormal results, use of population management strategies within clinical care settings is necessary to ensure that patients receive indicated follow-up. To facilitate tracking and management of cervical cancer screenings, clinical practices should take several steps:

1. Decide as a practice whether USPSTF, ACS, or ACOG screening guidelines will be followed.
2. Determine whether HPV primary screening, cotesting, or cytology-only screening will be performed.
3. Operationalize tracking systems for providers and patients to ensure that tests are performed when needed. This can use personnel, such as a dedicated nurse, to review and triage all cervical cancer screening results, or other methods, such as electronic health record prompts, or a combination of various tools.
4. Ensure that the strategy for population health management includes the goal of measuring and achieving high rates of recommended screening so that progress can be tracked.

Note that the ASCCP Risk-Based Management Consensus guidelines are the only national guidelines directing management of abnormal screening test results.[76] These guidelines give management recommendations for practices using primary HPV testing, cotesting, or cytology for screening. However, because cytology is substantially less sensitive than HPV testing for detecting precancer, cytology is recommended more frequently than HPV testing in follow-up of abnormal results. Specifically, cytology is recommended every 6 months when HPV testing or cotesting is recommended annually, and cytology is recommended annually when HPV testing or cotesting is recommended every 3 years. The increased frequency of required follow-up visits for 10% to 20% of the population may be an important factor when practices are considering the costs and benefits of different screening strategies. HPV testing or cotesting may be especially advantageous for practices whose patients are less able to comply with frequent follow-up visits, because negative HPV test results are more reassuring than negative cytology results and thus can be performed less frequently, allowing the clinical practices to focus their limited outreach resources on the highest-risk patients.

DISCUSSION
What Is the Most Effective Strategy for Cervical Cancer Prevention Throughout the Lifespan?

The most effective strategy for cervical cancer prevention evolves directly from understanding of the role of HPV in cervical carcinogenesis. Most oncogenic HPV infections are acquired between the ages of 18 and 26,[9] precancers peak between ages 25 and 35,[12] and cancer rates begin to rise at age 40 and remain elevated throughout the remaining years of life.[13,14] Thus primary prevention of HPV infections in adolescence followed by screening for and treatment of precancers in adults are the keys to cancer prevention.[26,79]

Ages 9 to 18

The first step is primary prevention: universal HPV vaccination of the current adolescent population. This is estimated to prevent up to 85% of cervical cancers, even in the absence of screening.[80]

Ages 18 to 24

Both screening and HPV vaccination are recommended for portions of this age group, yet neither is optimally effective. Because HPV infections accrue rapidly following sexual debut, HPV vaccine effectiveness decreases substantially when the series is initiated greater than ages 18 to 20.[28,29] However, although the prevalence of HPV infection is high in this age group, most infections and cervical lesions are destined to regress, such that treating precancers younger than age 25 is discouraged in all but the highest-risk cases.[76] Thus, this population derives limited benefit from screening. Screening guidelines universally state that the risks of screening outweigh benefits in immunocompetent individuals younger than age 21 years, and the 2020 ACS guidelines recommend initiating screening at age 25 years.[37,38,61,62]

Ages 25 to 65

All experts agree that screening is the key to cervical cancer prevention for this age group.[37,38,61,62] Experts also concur that clinical trials of HPV vaccination older than age 26 have demonstrated limited evidence for prevention of cervical cancer precursors; therefore, routine vaccination of this age group is not recommended.[30] Examination of the characteristics of cervical cancer screening tests conclusively demonstrate that HPV testing or cotesting detects more precancers per screening round than cytology screening alone.[48,49] Screening with HPV testing or cotesting can be performed less frequently than cytology alone with superior cancer prevention,[37,38,61,62] and HPV tests or cotests are preferred to cytology alone for surveillance following screening test abnormalities.[76] Cotesting detects approximately 5% more precancers per screening round than does HPV testing alone, but results in a substantial increase in cost and false-positive testing rates (defined as abnormal results that lead to additional diagnostic testing without detecting a precancer).[47,56,58] Data indicate that screening at ages 45 to 65 is crucial to preventing cancer among women older than age 65[73,74]; however, screening rates are low in this age group.[81] Therefore ensuring adequate screening at ages 45 to 65 should be an important goal of screening programs.

Ages 65 and Older

Individuals in this age group represent a conundrum in care. Although routine screening is not recommended,[47,56,58] they represent 20% of cervical cancers, and have excess mortality compared with younger women.[14,72] In addition, performing screening, diagnostic, and treatment procedures in individuals more than 10 years past menopause is more difficult and less likely to yield accurate results because of vaginal atrophy and, in some cases, physical mobility issues. Therefore, the key to preventing cervical cancer in individuals older than age 65 may be ensuring adequate screening at ages 45 to 65. Many patients who develop cervical cancer at age greater than 65 did not fulfill exit criteria before cessation of screening.[73,74] In contrast, the rate of cervical cancer following multiple rounds of HPV testing or cotesting is extremely low.[51] Yet, 12% to 18% of women age 45 to 65 report no cervical cancer screening in greater than 5 years.[82] Thus, encouraging women to engage in cervical cancer screening around and through the menopausal transition has the potential to dramatically decrease cancer rates older than age 65.

SUMMARY

Because of decades of important research on the relationship of HPV and cervical cancer, the tools are now in hand to prevent nearly all cases of the disease.[83] Cervical cancer prevention is no longer "one size fits all" with annual examinations for all adult women. Primary prevention of cervical cancer begins in adolescence with universal vaccination to prevent infection with HPV in the future. Most adults have been exposed to oncogenic HPV, therefore secondary prevention with screening becomes the primary mode of prevention for adults. The increased precision afforded by incorporating HPV testing into screening algorithms allows providers and healthcare systems to focus resources on high-risk individuals and reduce unnecessary screening and diagnostic procedures in low-risk individuals. This is efficient and effective, but requires investment of time and resources into the development of robust population management systems to appropriately track and recall patients for needed screenings and interventions. Finally, cervical cancer continues to occur most frequently in unscreened and underscreened patients, so ensuring that all adolescents receive HPV vaccinations and that all adults with a cervix receive screening and follow-up are most crucial to decreasing rates of cervical cancer.

DISCLOSURE

No disclosures.

REFERENCES

1. SEER. Available at: http://seer.cancer.gov/statfacts/html/cervix.html#incidence-mortality. Accessed April 21, 2020.
2. Schiffman M, Wentzensen N, Wacholder S, et al. Human papillomavirus testing in the prevention of cervical cancer. J Natl Cancer Inst 2011;103(5):368–83.
3. Clifford G, Franceschi S, Diaz M, et al. Chapter 3: HPV type-distribution in women with and without cervical neoplastic diseases. Vaccine 2006;24(Suppl 3):S26–34.
4. Schiffman MH, Brinton LA. The epidemiology of cervical carcinogenesis. Cancer 1995;76(10 Suppl):1888–901.
5. Demarco M, Egemen D, Raine-Bennett TR, et al. A study of partial human papillomavirus genotyping in support of the 2019 ASCCP risk-based management consensus guidelines. J Low Genit Tract Dis 2020;24(2):144–7.
6. Ault KA. Epidemiology and natural history of human papillomavirus infections in the female genital tract. Infect Dis Obstet Gynecol 2006;14(1):40470.
7. McQuillan G, Kruszon-Moran D, Markowitz LE, et al. Prevalence of HPV in adults aged 18-69: United States, 2011-2014. NCHS Data Brief 2017;(280):1–8.
8. Winer RL, Lee SK, Hughes JP, et al. Genital human papillomavirus infection: incidence and risk factors in a cohort of female university students. Am J Epidemiol 2003;157(3):218–26.
9. Laprise J-F, Chesson HW, Markowitz LE, et al. Effectiveness and cost-effectiveness of human papillomavirus vaccination through age 45 years in the United States. Ann Intern Med 2019. https://doi.org/10.7326/M19-1182.

10. Rodríguez AC, Schiffman M, Herrero R, et al. Rapid clearance of human papillomavirus and implications for clinical focus on persistent infections. J Natl Cancer Inst 2008;100(7):513–7.

11. McCredie MRE, Sharples KJ, Paul C, et al. Natural history of cervical neoplasia and risk of invasive cancer in women with cervical intraepithelial neoplasia 3: a retrospective cohort study. Lancet Oncol 2008;9(5):425–34.

12. McClung NM, Gargano JW, Park IU, et al. Estimated number of cases of high-grade cervical lesions diagnosed among women—United States, 2008 and 2016. MMWR Morb Mortal Wkly Rep 2019;68(15):337–43.

13. Beavis AL, Gravitt PE, Rositch AF. Hysterectomy-corrected cervical cancer mortality rates reveal a larger racial disparity in the United States. Cancer 2017; 123(6):1044–50.

14. Feldman S, Cook E, Davis M, et al. Cervical cancer incidence among elderly women in Massachusetts compared with younger women. J Low Genit Tract Dis 2018;22(4):314–7.

15. Hariri S, Unger ER, Schafer S, et al. HPV type attribution in high-grade cervical lesions: assessing the potential benefits of vaccines in a population-based evaluation in the United States. Cancer Epidemiol Biomarkers Prev 2015;24(2):393–9.

16. Group FIS. Quadrivalent vaccine against human papillomavirus to prevent high-grade cervical lesions. N Engl J Med 2007;356(19):1915–27.

17. Oliver SE, Unger ER, Lewis R, et al. Prevalence of human papillomavirus among females after vaccine introduction: National Health and Nutrition Examination Survey, United States, 2003-2014. J Infect Dis 2017;216(5):594–603.

18. Drolet M, Benard E, Boily MC, et al. Population-level impact and herd effects following human papillomavirus vaccination programmes: a systematic review and meta-analysis. Lancet Infect Dis 2015;15(5):565–80.

19. Ali H, Donovan B, Wand H, et al. Genital warts in young Australians five years into national human papillomavirus vaccination programme: national surveillance data. BMJ 2013;346:f2032.

20. Brotherton JM, Fridman M, May CL, et al. Early effect of the HPV vaccination programme on cervical abnormalities in Victoria, Australia: an ecological study. Lancet 2011;377(9783):2085–92.

21. Gertig DM, Brotherton JM, Budd AC, et al. Impact of a population-based HPV vaccination program on cervical abnormalities: a data linkage study. BMC Med 2013;11:227.

22. Ueda Y, Yagi A, Nakayama T, et al. Dynamic changes in Japan's prevalence of abnormal findings in cervical cytology depending on birth year. Sci Rep 2018; 8(1):5612.

23. Dorton BJ, Vitonis AF, Feldman S. Comparing cervical cytology and histology among human papillomavirus-vaccinated and -unvaccinated women in an academic colposcopy clinic. Obstet Gynecol 2015;126(4):785–91.

24. Brogly SB, Perkins RB, Zepf D, et al. Human papillomavirus vaccination and cervical cytology in young minority women. Sex Transm Dis 2014;41(8):511–4.

25. Luostarinen T, Apter D, Dillner J, et al. Vaccination protects against invasive HPV-associated cancers. Int J Cancer 2018;142(10):2186–7.

26. Guo F, Cofie LE, Berenson AB. Cervical cancer incidence in young U.S. females after human papillomavirus vaccine introduction. Am J Prev Med 2018;55(2): 197–204.

27. Kjaer SK, Sigurdsson K, Iversen O-E, et al. A pooled analysis of continued prophylactic efficacy of quadrivalent human papillomavirus (types 6/11/16/18)

vaccine against high-grade cervical and external genital lesions. Cancer Prev Res (Phila) 2009;2(10):868–78.

28. Castle PE, Xie X, Xue X, et al. Impact of human papillomavirus vaccination on the clinical meaning of cervical screening results. Prev Med 2019;118:44–50.

29. Herweijer E, Sundström K, Ploner A, et al. Quadrivalent HPV vaccine effectiveness against high-grade cervical lesions by age at vaccination: a population-based study. Int J Cancer 2016;138(12):2867–74.

30. Meites E, Szilagyi PG, Chesson HW, et al. Human papillomavirus vaccination for adults: updated recommendations of the Advisory Committee on Immunization Practices. MMWR Morb Mortal Wkly Rep 2019;68(32):698–702.

31. Saslow D, Andrews KS, Manassaram-Baptiste D, et al. Human papillomavirus vaccination 2020 guideline update: American Cancer Society guideline adaptation. CA Cancer J Clin 2020;70:274–80.

32. Dickinson JA, Stankiewicz A, Popadiuk C, et al. Reduced cervical cancer incidence and mortality in Canada: national data from 1932 to 2006. BMC Public Health 2012;12:992.

33. Singh GK, Jemal A. Socioeconomic and racial/ethnic disparities in cancer mortality, incidence, and survival in the United States, 1950-2014: over six decades of changing patterns and widening inequalities. J Environ Public Health 2017;2017: 2819372.

34. Castle PE, Kinney WK, Cheung LC, et al. Why does cervical cancer occur in a state-of-the-art screening program? Gynecol Oncol 2017;146(3):546–53.

35. Wang J, Elfström KM, Andrae B, et al. Cervical cancer case-control audit: results from routine evaluation of a nationwide cervical screening program. Int J Cancer 2020;146(5):1230–40.

36. Torre LA, Siegel RL, Ward EM, et al. Global cancer incidence and mortality rates and trends: an update. Cancer Epidemiol Biomarkers Prev 2016;25(1):16–27.

37. Saslow D, Solomon D, Lawson HW, et al. American Cancer Society, American Society for Colposcopy and Cervical Pathology, and American Society for Clinical Pathology screening guidelines for the prevention and early detection of cervical cancer. Am J Clin Pathol 2012;137(4):516–42.

38. US Preventive Services Task Force, Curry SJ, Krist AH, Owens DK, et al. Screening for cervical cancer: US Preventive Services Task Force Recommendation Statement. JAMA 2018;320(7):674–86.

39. Nanda K, McCrory DC, Myers ER, et al. Accuracy of the Papanicolaou test in screening for and follow-up of cervical cytologic abnormalities: a systematic review. Ann Intern Med 2000;132(10):810–9.

40. Fahey MT, Irwig L, Macaskill P. Meta-analysis of Pap test accuracy. Am J Epidemiol 1995;141(7):680–9.

41. Sankaranarayanan R, Nene BM, Shastri SS, et al. HPV screening for cervical cancer in rural India. N Engl J Med 2009;360(14):1385–94.

42. Sawaya GF, McConnell KJ, Kulasingam SL, et al. Risk of cervical cancer associated with extending the interval between cervical-cancer screenings. N Engl J Med 2003;349(16):1501–9.

43. Arbyn M, Smith SB, Temin S, et al. Collaboration on self-sampling and HPV testing. Detecting cervical precancer and reaching underscreened women by using HPV testing on self samples: updated meta-analyses. BMJ 2018;363: k4823.

44. Asciutto KC, Ernstson A, Forslund O, et al. Self-sampling with HPV mRNA analyses from vagina and urine compared with cervical samples. J Clin Virol 2018; 101:69–73.

45. Arrossi S, Thouyaret L, Herrero R, et al. Effect of self-collection of HPV DNA offered by community health workers at home visits on uptake of screening for cervical cancer (the EMA study): a population-based cluster-randomised trial. Lancet Glob Health 2015;3(2):e85–94.

46. Castle PE, Rausa A, Walls T, et al. Comparative community outreach to increase cervical cancer screening in the Mississippi Delta. Prev Med 2011;52(6):452–5.

47. Schiffman M, Kinney WK, Cheung LC, et al. Relative performance of HPV and cytology components of cotesting in cervical screening. J Natl Cancer Inst 2017. https://doi.org/10.1093/jnci/djx225.

48. Gage JC, Schiffman M, Katki HA, et al. Reassurance against future risk of pre-cancer and cancer conferred by a negative human papillomavirus test. J Natl Cancer Inst 2014;106(8). https://doi.org/10.1093/jnci/dju153.

49. Elfstrom KM, Smelov V, Johansson ALV, et al. Long term duration of protective effect for HPV negative women: follow-up of primary HPV screening randomised controlled trial. BMJ 2014;348:g130.

50. Castle PE, Glass AG, Rush BB, et al. Clinical human papillomavirus detection forecasts cervical cancer risk in women over 18 years of follow-up. J Clin Oncol 2012;30(25):3044–50.

51. Castle PE, Kinney WK, Xue X, et al. Effect of several negative rounds of human papillomavirus and cytology co-testing on safety against cervical cancer: an observational cohort study. Ann Intern Med 2018;168(1):20–9.

52. Smith MA, Canfell K. Projected impact of HPV vaccination and primary HPV screening on cervical adenocarcinoma: example from Australia. Papillomavirus Res 2017;3:134–41.

53. Smith HO, Tiffany MF, Qualls CR, et al. The rising incidence of adenocarcinoma relative to squamous cell carcinoma of the uterine cervix in the United States: a 24-year population-based study. Gynecol Oncol 2000;78(2):97–105.

54. Bray F, Carstensen B, Møller H, et al. Incidence trends of adenocarcinoma of the cervix in 13 European countries. Cancer Epidemiol Biomarkers Prev 2005;14(9): 2191–9.

55. Ronco G, Giorgi-Rossi P, Carozzi F, et al. Efficacy of human papillomavirus testing for the detection of invasive cervical cancers and cervical intraepithelial neoplasia: a randomised controlled trial. Lancet Oncol 2010;11(3):249–57.

56. Egemen D, Cheung LC, Chen X, et al. Risk estimates supporting the 2019 ASCCP Risk-Based Management Consensus Guidelines. J Low Genit Tract Dis 2020;24(2):132–43.

57. Castle PE, Rodríguez AC, Burk RD, et al. Short term persistence of human papillomavirus and risk of cervical precancer and cancer: population based cohort study. BMJ 2009;339:b2569.

58. Arbyn M, Sasieni P, Meijer CJLM, et al. Chapter 9: clinical applications of HPV testing: a summary of meta-analyses. Vaccine 2006;24 Suppl 3. S3/78-89.

59. Austin RM, Onisko A, Zhao C. Enhanced detection of cervical cancer and pre-cancer through use of imaged liquid-based cytology in routine cytology and HPV cotesting. Am J Clin Pathol 2018;150(5):385–92.

60. Kim JJ, Burger EA, Regan C, et al. Screening for cervical cancer in primary care: a decision analysis for the U.S. Preventive services task force. Agency for Healthcare Research and Quality (US); 2018. Available at: http://www.ncbi.nlm.nih.gov/books/NBK525069/. Accessed April 9, 2019.

61. Committee on Practice Bulletins—Gynecology. Practice Bulletin No. 168: cervical cancer screening and prevention. Obstet Gynecol 2016;128(4):e111–30.

62. Fontham ET, Wolf AM, Church TR, et al. Cervical cancer screening for individuals at average risk: 2020 guideline update from the American Cancer Society. CA Cancer J Clin 2020. https://doi.org/10.3322/caac.21628.

63. Smith JS, Melendy A, Rana RK, et al. Age-specific prevalence of infection with human papillomavirus in females: a global review. J Adolesc Health 2008; 43(4):S5.e1-62.

64. Moscicki AB, Shiboski S, Broering J, et al. The natural history of human papillomavirus infection as measured by repeated DNA testing in adolescent and young women. J Pediatr 1998;132(2):277–84.

65. Schiffman M, Castle PE, Jeronimo J, et al. Human papillomavirus and cervical cancer. Lancet 2007;370(9590):890–907.

66. Bekos C, Schwameis R, Heinze G, et al. Influence of age on histologic outcome of cervical intraepithelial neoplasia during observational management: results from large cohort, systematic review, meta-analysis. Sci Rep 2018;8(1). https://doi.org/10.1038/s41598-018-24882-2.

67. McAllum B, Sykes PH, Sadler L, et al. Is the treatment of CIN 2 always necessary in women under 25 years old? Am J Obstet Gynecol 2011;205(5):478.e1-7.

68. Tainio K, Athanasiou A, Tikkinen KAO, et al. Clinical course of untreated cervical intraepithelial neoplasia grade 2 under active surveillance: systematic review and meta-analysis. BMJ 2018;360:k499.

69. Jakobsson M, Gissler M, Paavonen J, et al. Loop electrosurgical excision procedure and the risk for preterm birth. Obstet Gynecol 2009;114(3):504–10.

70. Sadler L, Saftlas A, Wang W, et al. Treatment for cervical intraepithelial neoplasia and risk of preterm delivery. JAMA 2004;291(17):2100–6.

71. Werner CL, Lo JY, Heffernan T, et al. Loop electrosurgical excision procedure and risk of preterm birth. Obstet Gynecol 2010;115(3):605–8.

72. Rositch AF, Nowak RG, Gravitt PE. Increased age and race-specific incidence of cervical cancer after correction for hysterectomy prevalence in the United States from 2000 to 2009. Cancer 2014;120(13):2032–8.

73. Dinkelspiel H, Fetterman B, Poitras N, et al. Screening history preceding a diagnosis of cervical cancer in women age 65 and older. Gynecol Oncol 2012;126(2): 203–6.

74. Castañón A, Landy R, Cuzick J, et al. Cervical screening at age 50-64 years and the risk of cervical cancer at age 65 years and older: population-based case control study. PLoS Med 2014;11(1):e1001585.

75. Boulanger JC, Gondry J, Verhoest P, et al. Treatment of CIN after menopause. Eur J Obstet Gynecol Reprod Biol 2001;95(2):175–80.

76. Perkins RB, Guido RS, Castle PE, et al. 2019 ASCCP risk-based management consensus guidelines for abnormal cervical cancer screening tests and cancer precursors. J Low Genit Tract Dis 2020;24(2):102–31.

77. Fetters MD, Fischer G, Reed BD. Effectiveness of vaginal Papanicolaou smear screening after total hysterectomy for benign disease. JAMA 1996;275(12): 940–7.

78. Sirovich BE, Welch HG. The frequency of Pap smear screening in the United States. J Gen Intern Med 2004;19(3):243–50.

79. Spence AR, Goggin P, Franco EL. Process of care failures in invasive cervical cancer: systematic review and meta-analysis. Prev Med 2007;45(2–3):93–106.

80. Joura EA, Ault KA, Bosch FX, et al. Attribution of 12 high-risk human papillomavirus genotypes to infection and cervical disease. Cancer Epidemiol Biomarkers Prev 2014;23(10):1997–2008.

81. Harper DM, Plegue M, Harmes KM, et al. Three large scale surveys highlight the complexity of cervical cancer under-screening among women 45–65 years of age in the United States. Prev Med 2020;130:105880.

82. White MC, Shoemaker ML, Benard VB. Cervical cancer screening and incidence by age: unmet needs near and after the stopping age for screening. Am J Prev Med 2017;53(3):392–5.

83. Lippman SM, Abate-Shen C, Colbert Maresso KL, et al. AACR White Paper: Shaping the Future of Cancer Prevention - A Roadmap for Advancing Science and Public Health. Cancer Prev Res (Phila) 2018;11(12):735–78.

UNITED STATES POSTAL SERVICE ®

Statement of Ownership, Management, and Circulation
(All Periodicals Publications Except Requester Publications)

1. Publication Title
MEDICAL CLINICS IN NORTH AMERICA

2. Publication Number
337 – 340

3. Filing Date
9/18/2020

4. Issue Frequency
JAN, MAR, MAY, JUL, SEP, NOV

5. Number of Issues Published Annually
6

6. Annual Subscription Price
$295.00

7. Complete Mailing Address of Known Office of Publication *(Not printer) (Street, city, county, state, and ZIP+4®)*
ELSEVIER INC.
230 Park Avenue, Suite 800
New York, NY 10169

Contact Person
STEPHEN R. BUSHING

Telephone *(Include area code)*
215-239-3688

8. Complete Mailing Address of Headquarters or General Business Office of Publisher *(Not printer)*
ELSEVIER INC.
230 Park Avenue, Suite 800
New York, NY 10169

9. Full Names and Complete Mailing Addresses of Publisher, Editor, and Managing Editor *(Do not leave blank)*

Publisher *(Name and complete mailing address)*
Dolores Meloni, ELSEVIER INC.
1600 JOHN F KENNEDY BLVD. SUITE 1800
PHILADELPHIA, PA 19103-2899

Editor *(Name and complete mailing address)*
KATERINA HEIDHAUSEN, ELSEVIER INC.
1600 JOHN F KENNEDY BLVD. SUITE 1800
PHILADELPHIA, PA 19103-2899

Managing Editor *(Name and complete mailing address)*
PATRICK MANLEY, ELSEVIER INC.
1600 JOHN F KENNEDY BLVD. SUITE 1800
PHILADELPHIA, PA 19103-2899

10. Owner *(Do not leave blank. If the publication is owned by a corporation, give the name and address of the corporation immediately followed by the names and addresses of all stockholders owning or holding 1 percent or more of the total amount of stock. If not owned by a corporation, give the names and addresses of the individual owners. If owned by a partnership or other unincorporated firm, give its name and address as well as those of each individual owner. If the publication is published by a nonprofit organization, give its name and address.)*

Full Name	Complete Mailing Address
WHOLLY OWNED SUBSIDIARY OF REED/ELSEVIER, US HOLDINGS	1600 JOHN F KENNEDY BLVD. SUITE 1800 PHILADELPHIA, PA 19103-2899

11. Known Bondholders, Mortgagees, and Other Security Holders Owning or Holding 1 Percent or More of Total Amount of Bonds, Mortgages, or Other Securities. If none, check box ▶ ☐ None

Full Name	Complete Mailing Address
N/A	

12. Tax Status *(For completion by nonprofit organizations authorized to mail at nonprofit rates) (Check one)*
The purpose, function, and nonprofit status of this organization and the exempt status for federal income tax purposes:
☒ Has Not Changed During Preceding 12 Months
☐ Has Changed During Preceding 12 Months *(Publisher must submit explanation of change with this statement)*

PS Form **3526**, July 2014 *(Page 1 of 4 (see instructions page 4))* PSN: 7530-01-000-9931 PRIVACY NOTICE: See our privacy policy on www.usps.com

---

13. Publication Title
MEDICAL CLINICS IN NORTH AMERICA

14. Issue Date for Circulation Data Below
JULY 2020

15. Extent and Nature of Circulation

		Average No. Copies Each Issue During Preceding 12 Months	No. Copies of Single Issue Published Nearest to Filing Date
a. Total Number of Copies *(Net press run)*		452	392
b. Paid Circulation *(By Mail and Outside the Mail)*	(1) Mailed Outside-County Paid Subscriptions Stated on PS Form 3541 (Include paid distribution above nominal rate, advertiser's proof copies, and exchange copies)	265	234
	(2) Mailed In-County Paid Subscriptions Stated on PS Form 3541 (Include paid distribution above nominal rate, advertiser's proof copies, and exchange copies)	0	0
	(3) Paid Distribution Outside the Mails Including Sales Through Dealers and Carriers, Street Vendors, Counter Sales, and Other Paid Distribution Outside USPS®	129	116
	(4) Paid Distribution by Other Classes of Mail Through the USPS (e.g., First-Class Mail®)	0	0
c. Total Paid Distribution *(Sum of 15b (1), (2), (3), and (4))*	▶	394	350
d. Free or Nominal Rate Distribution *(By Mail and Outside the Mail)*	(1) Free or Nominal Rate Outside-County Copies included on PS Form 3541	39	27
	(2) Free or Nominal Rate In-County Copies Included on PS Form 3541	0	0
	(3) Free or Nominal Rate Copies Mailed at Other Classes Through the USPS (e.g., First-Class Mail)	0	0
	(4) Free or Nominal Rate Distribution Outside the Mail (Carriers or other means)	0	0
e. Total Free or Nominal Rate Distribution *(Sum of 15d (1), (2), (3) and (4))*	▶	39	27
f. Total Distribution *(Sum of 15c and 15e)*	▶	433	377
g. Copies not Distributed *(See Instructions to Publishers #4 (page #3))*	▶	19	15
h. Total *(Sum of 15f and g)*	▶	452	392
i. Percent Paid *(15c divided by 15f times 100)*	▶	90.99%	92.83%

* If you are claiming electronic copies, go to line 16 on page 3. If you are not claiming electronic copies, skip to line 17 on page 3.

16. Electronic Copy Circulation

	Average No. Copies Each Issue During Preceding 12 Months	No. Copies of Single Issue Published Nearest to Filing Date
a. Paid Electronic Copies ▶		
b. Total Paid Print Copies (Line 15c) + Paid Electronic Copies (Line 16a) ▶		
c. Total Print Distribution (Line 15f) + Paid Electronic Copies (Line 16a) ▶		
d. Percent Paid (Both Print & Electronic Copies) (16b divided by 16c × 100) ▶		

☒ I certify that 50% of all my distributed copies (electronic and print) are paid above a nominal price.

17. Publication of Statement of Ownership
☒ If the publication is a general publication, publication of this statement is required. Will be printed in the NOVEMBER 2020 issue of this publication. ☐ Publication not required.

18. Signature and Title of Editor, Publisher, Business Manager, or Owner
Malathi Samayan *(signature)*

Malathi Samayan - Distribution Controller

Date 9/18/2020

I certify that all information furnished on this form is true and complete. I understand that anyone who furnishes false or misleading information on this form or who omits material or information requested on the form may be subject to criminal sanctions (including fines and imprisonment) and/or civil sanctions (including civil penalties).

PS Form **3526**, July 2014 *(Page 3 of 4)* PRIVACY NOTICE: See our privacy policy on www.usps.com

Moving?

Make sure your subscription moves with you!

To notify us of your new address, find your **Clinics Account Number** (located on your mailing label above your name), and contact customer service at:

Email: **journalscustomerservice-usa@elsevier.com**

800-654-2452 (subscribers in the U.S. & Canada)
314-447-8871 (subscribers outside of the U.S. & Canada)

Fax number: 314-447-8029

Elsevier Health Sciences Division
Subscription Customer Service
3251 Riverport Lane
Maryland Heights, MO 63043

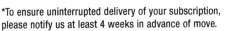

*To ensure uninterrupted delivery of your subscription, please notify us at least 4 weeks in advance of move.

ELSEVIER

Printed and bound by CPI Group (UK) Ltd, Croydon, CR0 4YY

03/10/2024

01040477-0015